Oxygen

Creating
a New Paradigm

Oxygen

Creating a New Paradigm

Paul L. Marino, MD, PhD

Clinical Associate Professor
Weill Cornell Medical College
New York, New York

Illustrations by Patricia Gast

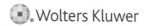. Wolters Kluwer

Philadelphia · Baltimore · New York · London
Buenos Aires · Hong Kong · Sydney · Tokyo

Senior Acquisitions Editor: Keith Donnellan
Senior Development Editor: Ashley Fischer
Marketing Manager: Kirsten Watrud
Production Project Manager: David Saltzberg
Design Coordinator: Stephen Druding
Illustrator: Patricia Gast
Manufacturing Coordinator: Beth Welsh
Prepress Vendor: TNQ Technologies

9 8 7 6 5 4 3 2 1

Printed in the United States of America

Library of Congress Cataloging-in-Publication Data

ISBN-13: 978-1-4963-9484-2

Cataloging in Publication data available on request from publisher.

This work is provided "as is," and the publisher disclaims any and all warranties, express or implied, including any warranties as to accuracy, comprehensiveness, or currency of the content of this work.

This work is no substitute for individual patient assessment based upon healthcare professionals' examination of each patient and consideration of, among other things, age, weight, gender, current or prior medical conditions, medication history, laboratory data and other factors unique to the patient. The publisher does not provide medical advice or guidance and this work is merely a reference tool. Healthcare professionals, and not the publisher, are solely responsible for the use of this work including all medical judgments and for any resulting diagnosis and treatments.

Given continuous, rapid advances in medical science and health information, independent professional verification of medical diagnoses, indications, appropriate pharmaceutical selections and dosages, and treatment options should be made and healthcare professionals should consult a variety of sources. When prescribing medication, healthcare professionals are advised to consult the product information sheet (the manufacturer's package insert) accompanying each drug to verify, among other things, conditions of use, warnings and side effects and identify any changes in dosage schedule or contraindications, particularly if the medication to be administered is new, infrequently used or has a narrow therapeutic range. To the maximum extent permitted under applicable law, no responsibility is assumed by the publisher for any injury and/or damage to persons or property, as a matter of products liability, negligence law or otherwise, or from any reference to or use by any person of this work.

shop.lww.com

MPP0921

To my son,
Daniel Joseph Marino.
Now a man …
but always my boy.

The secret of science is to ask the right question …

Sir Henry Tizard
(1885-1959)

Preface

> "Scientific revolutions are inaugurated by a growing sense…
> that an existing paradigm has ceased to function adequately."
>
> Thomas Kuhn, 1962 (1)

Thomas Kuhn (1922-1996) is considered one of the most influential voices in the philosophy of science in the 20th century. Kuhn is an American who began his career with a PhD in physics, but soon thereafter changed his focus to the philosophy and history of science. In 1962, he published his signature work, *The Structure of Scientific Revolutions* (1), which describes his concept of how science progresses. This concept is summarized as follows. Each specialty or discipline in science adopts a model or *paradigm* to describe the theoretical or practical observations in that discipline. The scientific activity within each discipline is then based on the predictions of the prevailing paradigm, with little or no attempt to question the validity of the paradigm. When experimental observations are not consistent with the predictions of the paradigm, the validity of the observation (not the paradigm) is questioned. Only after repeated instances in which observations are at odds with the prevailing paradigm is there a shift in focus to a critical evaluation of the paradigm. This eventually leads to a change, or *paradigm shift*, that provides a better fit with the experimental observations.

Kuhn's description of how science progresses seems to apply to the current paradigm for oxygen. There is an unquestioned obeisance to oxygen as the *sine qua non* for life on this planet, and promoting tissue oxygenation is considered equivalent to promoting life. The strength of this belief is demonstrated in the case of the pulmonary artery catheter: i.e., when clinical studies showed that increasing O_2 delivery with pulmonary artery catheters did not improve survival, the catheter was blamed (and largely abandoned), while the possibility that an increase on O_2 delivery does not improve survival was never entertained.

What is neglected in the popular view of oxygen is its destructive nature; i.e., oxygen disrupts organic molecules (via oxidation), and this process can damage all vital cell components and produce a lethal form of cell injury. In fact, a wealth of evidence has accumulated over the past 50 years showing that oxygen (oxidation) is a *source* of pathological injury in a multitude of diseases. This destructive side of oxygen has been neglected in clinical medicine, and it deserves more attention. This book provides that attention, and reevaluates some traditional concepts about how the human body is designed in relation to oxygen, and how oxygen should be used in clinical practice.

This book employs a series of questions to examine or illuminate a specific feature related to oxygen. There are two major sections in the book. The first section, titled "How Important is Oxygen?," debunks some of the traditional beliefs about oxygen, and the practices used to promote tissue oxygenation. The first two chapters examine the importance of O_2 delivery in the functional role of the heart, lungs, and the erythron (the red blood cell-hemoglobin unit), and the information presented demonstrates that, in each case, the transport and elimination of CO_2 takes precedence over O_2 delivery. The third chapter looks at the distribution of O_2 in the human body, and reveals that there is a paucity of O_2 in tissues, and that aerobic metabolism is designed to operate in such an environment. The fourth chapter examines the common belief that tissue hypoxia is the final common pathway in the death of aerobic organisms, and shows that there is little evidence to support this belief. The last two chapters in the section examine two common practices used to promote tissue oxygenation (i.e., oxygen therapy and red blood cell transfusions) and reveals a lack of evidence that either of these practices achieves it goal. Furthermore, each of these interventions elicits a countermeasure (e.g., oxygen produces vasoconstriction) that helps to maintain the low-O_2 environment in tissues. Limiting exposure of the vital organs to oxygen will limit the risk of oxidative tissue injury, which gives a teleological purpose to the oxygen-poor interior of the human body.

The second section of the book, titled "How Destructive is Oxygen?," focuses on the damaging effects of oxygen (oxidation). Individual chapters in this section describe the general effects of oxidation (Chapter 7), the production of "reactive oxygen species" (ROS) and the mechanisms of oxidative cell injury (Chapter 8), and the participation of ROS in the inflammatory response (Chapter 9), radiation injury (Chapter 10), and aging (Chapter 11). Additional chapters describe antioxidant protection (Chapter 12) and the importance of antioxidant protection in hyperoxic lung injury (Chapter 13).

The final chapter in the book summarizes the relevant information presented throughout the book, which creates the conceptual view that *oxygen is a destructive molecule, and the human body is designed to protect the vital organs from the damaging effects of oxygen.* This is diametrically opposed to the current belief that flooding the tissues with oxygen is necessary for promoting life, and it indicates that *patient management should have an "oxygen-protective", rather than an "oxygen-promoting", design.* Recommendations for this oxygen-protective strategy are presented in the final chapter of the book.

Oxygen has the unique ability to decompose organic matter, which is why food is stored in vacuum-sealed containers, and why we use cellophane wrapping and tightly-sealed plastic containers to keep food "fresh". Since we protect the organic matter in our food from oxygen, we should do the same for the organic matter in our patients.

1. Kuhn TS. The Structure of Scientific Revolutions. Chicago: University of Chicago Press, 1962.

Acknowledgments

To my editor and friend, Keith Donnellan, for his PATIENCE and guidance in completing this work. Keith is the type of editor that every author should have. And to Ashley Fischer, development editor at Wolters Kluwer, whose efficiency and kind manner did not go unnoticed. And finally, to my longtime associate, Patricia Gast, who did the page layouts and illustrations for this book. This is our fifth book together, and none of them would have seen the light of day without her.

Table of Contents

How Important is Oxygen?

Is O_2 delivery the principal function of the cardiorespiratory system?

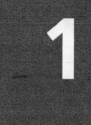

1

> "The purpose of the cardiorespiratory system is to deliver adequate amounts of oxygen to meet tissue demand."
>
> Adolph Fick, 1870

One of the traditional perceptions in the "oxygen mythos" is the notion that the heart and lungs are dedicated primarily to the task of delivering oxygen to the tissues. However, there is more than a "supply side" to energy conversion processes like metabolism (as we all know by witnessing the rise in atmospheric CO_2 levels), and the following presentation will demonstrate that the cardiorespiratory system is more concerned with removing metabolic waste (i.e., CO_2) than delivering oxygen.

VENTILATION

Control of Ventilation

In 1905, John Scott Haldane and John Giles Priestley published a landmark study on the control of ventilation (1). Using themselves as the test subjects, these investigators reported the following three observations: 1) The CO_2 pressure (PCO_2) in alveolar gas is remarkably constant when atmospheric pressure is varied, while the O_2 pressure (PO_2) varies widely. 2) Alveolar ventilation (in L/min) is exquisitely sensitive to changes in alveolar PCO_2: e.g., an increase in alveolar PCO_2 of just 0.2% (or 1.5 mm Hg) results in a 100% increase in alveolar ventilation. 3) There is no ventilatory response to a decrease in inspired O_2 until the O_2 pressure drops below 13% of atmospheric pressure. The conclusion from these observations was stated as follows: "The regulation of alveolar ventilation in breathing depends, under normal conditions, exclusively on the CO_2 pressure in the respiratory centre." This conclusion about the primacy of CO_2 in the control of ventilation is one of the cornerstones of respiratory physiology.

The ventilatory responses to CO_2 and O_2 are shown for comparison in Figure 1.1. The CO_2 response curve on the left shows a linear ventilatory response to changes in arterial PCO_2 ($PaCO_2$), with a slope of approximately 2 L/min/mm Hg when the arterial PO_2 is held at normal levels (2). Although not shown, this response continues until the $PaCO_2$ approaches 100 mm Hg, and thereafter elevations in $PaCO_2$ depress ventilation (and also depress consciousness). The intersection of the CO_2 response curve with the horizontal dotted line identifies the $PaCO_2$ associated with a normal level of ventilation (6 L/min in this case). The portion of the line below the normal $PaCO_2$ identifies hypocapnia as a cause of hypoventilation. (*Note:* Hypometabolism is the only source of hypocapnia that is independent of ventilation.) In contrast to the CO_2 response curve, the O_2 response curve (on the right in Figure 1.1) has a hyperbolic contour and shows no ventilatory response until the arterial PO_2 (PaO_2) drops to about 60 mm Hg (2). Of interest, there are otherwise healthy individuals who have no ventilatory response to hypoxemia when the $PaCO_2$ is normal (3), and this has no apparent adverse consequences (at least in the absence of hypoxemia). In fact, a PaO_2 of 60–90 mm Hg is the range encountered in almost all individuals at sea level (even those with advanced lung disease, who are given supplemental O_2 when the PaO_2 falls below 60 mm Hg), so the ventilatory response to hypoxemia has little or no relevance in everyday life.

Comparison of the O_2 and CO_2 response curves clearly shows the primacy of CO_2 over O_2 in the control of ventilation. Stated another way, *the ventilatory apparatus is designed primarily to eliminate CO_2*, which is the principal byproduct of metabolism. The ventilatory response to CO_2 is mediated by specialized neurons in the lower brainstem (called "chemoreceptors") that are distinct from the periodically firing neurons that generate automatic breathing (4). The ventilatory response to low O_2 is mediated by more peripherally placed chemoreceptors in the carotid body, which is located at the bifurcation of the common carotid artery on either side of the neck (near the carotid baroreceptors), and is innervated by the glossopharyngeal nerve (cranial nerve IX). The placement of these chemoreceptors for CO_2 and O_2 (i.e., central vs peripheral) also suggests a more primitive role for CO_2.

The Abundance of CO_2

A comparison of the total volumes of O_2 and CO_2 in the blood, as shown in Table 1.1, reveals a relative abundance of CO_2. (It also reveals the paucity of O_2 in the blood; i.e., the 820 mL of O_2 in the blood is enough to support aerobic metabolism for only 3½ minutes when the resting O_2 consumption is a typical 250 mL/min.

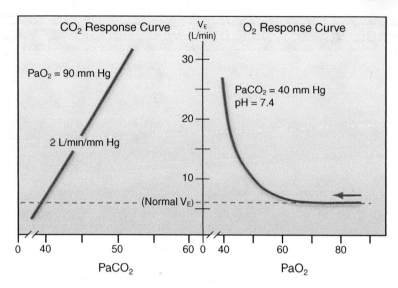

FIGURE 1.1 Ventilatory responses to changes in arterial PCO₂ (PaCO₂) and arterial PO₂ (PaO₂). VE is exhaled volume (in liters) per minute. Horizontal dotted line indicates the normal VE (6 L/min). Curves redrawn from Reference 2. See text for further explanation.

For more on this issue, see Chapter 3.) CO_2 is much more soluble in aqueous fluids than O_2, but dissolved CO_2 represents only 5% of the total CO_2 in blood (5). The major reason for the abundance of CO_2 over O_2 is the tendency for CO_2 to react with water and produce carbonic acid (H_2CO_3), which rapidly dissociates into hydrogen ions (H+) and bicarbonate ions (HCO_3^-), as shown below:

$$CO_2 + H_2O \rightarrow H_2CO_3 \rightarrow H^+ + HCO3^- \qquad (1.1)$$

The "CO₂ hydration" reaction normally requires 40 seconds for completion, but in the presence of the enzyme *carbonic anhydrase,* the reaction is completed in less than 10 milliseconds (6). Carbonic anhydrase is confined to red blood cells, so the CO_2 in plasma enters the red blood cell and is rapidly hydrated to generate H^+ (which is buffered by hemoglobin) and HCO_3^- (which is extruded back into the plasma). The rapid hydration reaction creates an "erythrocyte sink" that accommodates large volumes of CO_2.

Table 1.1   Oxygen and Carbon Dioxide in Blood

	Arterial	Venous	Total
Blood Volume	1.25 L	3.75 L	5.0 L
O_2 Content[1] Total O_2	200 mL/L 250 mL	152 mL/L 570 mL	 820 mL
CO_2 Content[2] Total CO_2	490 mL/L 613 mL	530 mL/L 1,988 mL	 2,601 mL

[1]See Chapter 3 for the derivation of this O_2 content.
[2]From Reference 5.

(*Note:* The ability of aqueous fluids to hold large volumes of CO_2, especially at high pressures, is the basis for "carbonation." Anyone who has shaken a bottle of champagne and then popped the cork has witnessed how much CO_2 can be held in aqueous fluids.)

Acid Excretion by the Lungs

The elimination of CO_2 by the lungs can be quantified using a modified Fick equation: i.e.,

$$VCO_2 = CO \ \times \ (CvCO_2 - CaCO_2) \qquad (1.2)$$

where VCO_2 is the rate of CO_2 elimination by the lungs (in mL/min), CO is the cardiac output (in L/min), and $(CvCO_2 - CaCO_2)$ is the difference in CO_2 content between venous and arterial blood (in mL/L). The components of this equation are illustrated in Figure 1.2. Using a cardiac output of 6 L/min, and the $CvCO_2$ and $CaCO_2$ listed in Table 1.1, the VCO_2 is calculated as follows:

$$\begin{aligned} VCO_2 &= \ 6 \text{ L/min} \ \times \ (530 - 490) \text{ mL/L} \qquad (1.3) \\ &= 240 \text{ mL/min} \end{aligned}$$

Since CO_2 exists as an acid (carbonic acid) in aqueous fluids, the VCO_2 can also be expressed as a rate of acid excretion. To accomplish this, the CO_2 content must be expressed as the concentration of a dissociable acid: i.e., in mEq/L. The conversion from mL/L to mEq/L is based on the fact that 1 mole (or 1 Equivalent) of a substance occupies a volume of 22.3 liters, so 1 mmol (or 1 mEq) of the substance has a volume of 22.3 mL.

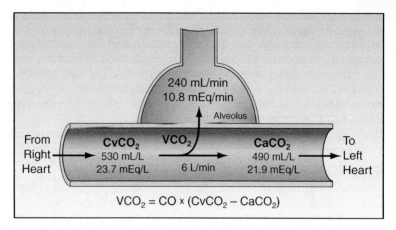

FIGURE 1.2 The rate of CO_2 elimination in the lungs (VCO_2), expressed as a volume of gas (in mL/min) and as excretion of an acid (in mEq/min). The cardiac output (CO) is indicated as 6 L/min, and the $CvCO_2$ and $CaCO_2$ represent the CO_2 content in venous and arterial blood, respectively. See text for further explanation.

Therefore:

$$CO_2 \text{ Content (mL/L)} / 22.3 = CO_2 \text{ Content (mEq/L)} \quad (1.4)$$

If Equation 1.3 is recalculated using the $CvCO_2$ and $CaCO_2$ expressed in mEq/L, the derived VCO_2 is the rate of acid excretion by the lungs (in mEq/min): i.e.,

$$VCO_2 = 6 \text{ L/min} \times (23.7 - 21.9) \text{ mEq/L} \quad (1.5)$$
$$= 10.8 \text{ mEq/min}$$

The daily acid excretion by the lungs is then $10.8 \times 1440 = 15,552$ mEq. In comparison, the daily acid excretion by the kidneys is only 40–80 mEq (5). This means that *the major organ of acid excretion in the human body is the lungs, not the kidneys.*

CIRCULATION

Control of Cardiac Output

One of the fundamental tenets of cardiovascular physiology is *Starling's Law of the Heart* (an eponymous tribute to its originator, Ernest Starling) (7), which states that the strength of cardiac contractions is directly related the volume in the ventricles at the end of diastole. This is similar to the length-tension relationship in skeletal muscle, and the underlying mechanism is related to cross-bridging between contractile filaments in the myocytes. An increase in ventricular end-diastolic volume stretches cardiac myocytes to a new resting length, and this moves actin filaments into the narrow spaces between myosin filaments. This increases the number cross-bridges formed between the contractile (actin and myosin) filaments during muscle contraction, which then increases the force of contraction during systole.

Venous Return

Although cardiac filling during diastole is the determining factor for cardiac stroke output, cardiac filling is a reflection of the rate of venous return to the heart, and venous return is typically identified as the cardiac output controller (8). This is demonstrated in the following statement by Ernest Starling: "the output of the heart... is determined by the amount of blood flowing into the heart" (7). The role of venous return as the cardiac output controller can be confusing because, during steady-state conditions, venous return *is* the cardiac output (with the exception of the blood that flows from the bronchial arteries directly into the pulmonary circulation, which represents about 1–3% of the cardiac output). However, venous return does more than provide the volume for the cardiac output because it also determines the strength of ventricular contraction (by the mechanism just described). Thus, if volume is infused to increase venous return, the resulting increase in cardiac contractile strength (and hence cardiac stroke output) allows the circulatory system to adjust to the increment in intravascular volume, and it prevents venous congestion and unwanted edema formation.

In contrast to the role of venous return, there are no forces on the arterial side of the circulation that act as a cardiac output controller. In fact, the lack of a cardiac output response to changes in blood pressure is what prompted Ernest Starling to begin the experiments that identified cardiac filling as the controlling force for cardiac output (7). It is important to emphasize (at least for this presentation) that cardiac output is controlled from the venous side of the circulation (where CO_2 removal takes place), and not from the arterial side (where O_2 delivery takes place).

Implications

Considering that ventilation is controlled by CO_2 (a major end-product of metabolism), and cardiac output is controlled by the venous side of the circulation, it is possible to conclude that

CHAPTER 1 • Is O₂ delivery the principal function of the cardiorespiratory system?

9

the principal concern of the cardiorespiratory system is to eliminate metabolic waste (especially CO_2), and not to deliver O_2 to the tissues.

O₂ Delivery vs CO₂ Removal

The following approach provides further evidence of the primacy of CO_2 removal over O_2 delivery.

The rate of O_2 delivery (DO_2) in arterial blood is equivalent to the product of the cardiac output (CO) and the O_2 concentration (also called O_2 content) in arterial blood (CaO_2):

$$DO_2 = CO \times CaO_2 \qquad (1.6)$$

Using a CO of 6 L/min and a CaO_2 of 200 mL/L (from Table 1.1) yields a DO_2 of 1,200 mL/min (or 1.2 L/min). Thus, the DO_2 represents 20% of the cardiac output.

The cardiac output does not just deliver O_2 to tissues, it also removes the CO_2 produced by metabolism. The rate of CO_2 removal (RCO_2) in venous blood is equivalent to the product of the cardiac output (CO) and the CO_2 content in venous blood ($CvCO_2$):

$$RCO_2 = CO \times CvCO_2 \qquad (1.7)$$

Using the same CO of 6 L/min and a $CvCO_2$ of 530 mL/L (from Table 1.1) yields an RCO_2 of 3,180 mL/min (or 3.18 L/min). The RCO_2 thus represents 53% of the cardiac output, and it is more than 2.5 times the DO_2: i.e.,

$$RCO_2 / DO_2 = 2.65 \qquad (1.8)$$

The primacy of CO_2 removal over O_2 delivery is demonstrated in Figure 1.3, which shows the comparative effects of an increase in cardiac output (from 6 to 8 L/min) on the DO_2 and RCO_2. As predicted by Equation 1.8, the increase in RCO_2 is 2.65 times greater than the increase in DO_2. Note also that the increase in RCO_2 represents about 50% of the increase in cardiac output, while the increment in DO_2 is only 20% of the increment in cardiac output.

Implications

The relationships in Equation 1.6 are the basis for the common practice of promoting cardiac output to augment O_2 delivery in patients with advanced cardiac failure and circulatory shock. However, as demonstrated in the prior section, increasing the cardiac output does not specifically increase O_2 delivery. In fact, Figure 1.3 demonstrates that only 20% of an increment in cardiac output is dedicated to promoting O_2 delivery ($\Delta DO_2 = 0.2 \times \Delta CO$).

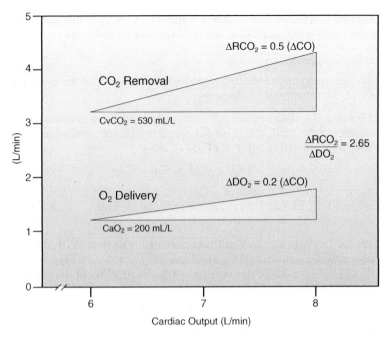

FIGURE 1.3 The comparative effects of an increase in cardiac output (CO) on the rates of CO_2 removal (RCO_2) and oxygen delivery (DO_2). The CaO_2 is the O_2 content in arterial blood, and the $CvCO_2$ is the CO_2 content in venous blood.

This means that, *when cardiac output is increased as a means of increasing O_2 delivery, most of the increment in cardiac output is doing other things,* and these "other things" can be beneficial (e.g., promoting CO_2 removal) or detrimental (e.g., promoting the spread of inflammatory cytokines).

The nonspecific relationship between cardiac output and O_2 delivery invalidates the conclusions of the numerous studies that have focused on the impact of promoting O_2 delivery (usually by promoting cardiac output) on clinical outcomes.

Circulatory Design

Anatomy textbooks invariably depict the arterial and venous systems as equivalent in size and capacity, but this is far from reality. The volume distribution in Table 1.2 indicates that about 75% of the blood volume is in the venous system, while the arterial side of the circulation contains only about 15% of the blood volume (9). The small cross-sectional areas and high flow velocities on the arterial side of the circulation indicate that the arterial circulation creates high-velocity "jets" of blood that reach the capillaries quickly. (This is similar to what happens when you tighten the nozzle on a garden hose, and is known as "Bernoulli principle.") Once the blood is in the capillaries, the large cross-sectional area is designed to promote exchange between tissues and blood. When the blood leaves the capillaries, it enters a large-volume, low-velocity venous system that acts as a reservoir for the continuous spillage of metabolic waste products. The benefits of a large-volume venous reservoir can be viewed in terms of CO_2 removal. As mentioned previously, CO_2 is removed in venous blood by reacting it with water (see Equation 1.1). The large volume of the (aqueous) venous reservoir then creates a sink that promotes the continued movement of CO_2 out of the tissues, and it provides enough substrate to accommodate the marked increases in CO_2 production that occur during exercise.

Table 1.2	Design of the Systemic Circulation*			
Segment	**Blood Volume**		**Cross-Sectional Area (m²)**	**Flow Velocity (cm/sec)**
	(mL)	**(%)**		
Aorta	565	14.3	50	40
Arteries			70	38
Arterioles	57	1.4	90	37
Capillaries	282	7.1	520	
Venules			260	8
Veins	3,048	77.2	130	12
Vena Cava			40	14

*Data for a total blood volume of 5.6 liters. Does not include the pulmonary circulation or blood in the heart chambers. Adapted from Reference 9.

A Familiar Example

The dangers of limited-capacity CO_2 removal were witnessed during the dramatic events of the Apollo 13 mission to the moon (10). An oxygen tank explosion in the command module forced the three astronauts into the smaller lunar module, and aborted the planned moon landing. During the return to Earth, there was a dangerous buildup of CO_2 in the lunar module, which was not equipped with CO_2 scrubbers large enough to remove the exhaled CO_2 from three astronauts. (A CO_2 scrubber is a device that removes CO_2 by combining it with a chemical substrate, similar to the removal of CO_2 in venous blood.) Thanks to the efforts of NASA engineers, the larger CO_2 scrubbers from the command module were adapted for use in the lunar module, thereby allowing the astronauts to return safely to Earth.

SUMMATION

The following information is used to show that the cardiorespiratory system is more concerned with removing CO_2 (the principal end-product of metabolism) than delivering O_2.

1. The principal controller of ventilation is CO_2, not O_2.
2. Because CO_2 is rapidly hydrated to form carbonic acid, the blood holds almost three times more CO_2 than O_2, and if CO_2 is expressed as an acid (in mEq), the lungs can be seen as the major organ of acid excretion in the body.
3. Cardiac output is controlled from the venous side of the circulation (where CO_2 removal takes place), and not from the arterial side (where O_2 delivery takes place).
4. Only 20% of the cardiac output is involved in O_2 delivery, whereas about 50% is involved in CO_2 removal.
5. For any given increment in cardiac output, the increase in CO_2 removal is 2.6 times greater than the increase in O_2 delivery.
6. About 75% of the blood volume is located on the venous side of the circulation, and this large-volume venous system acts as a reservoir for the continuous spillage of CO_2 and other metabolic waste products, and is capable of accommodating the marked increase in production of metabolic waste during exercise.

REFERENCES

1. Haldane JS, Priestley JG. The regulation of the lung-ventilation. J Physiol 1905; 32: 225-266.

2. Nunn JF. Control of breathing. In: Nunn's Applied Respiratory Physiology, 4th ed. Oxford: Butterworth-Heinemann, 1993:90-116.

3. Cormack RS, Cunningham DJC, Gee JBL. The effect of carbon dioxide on the respiratory response to want of oxygen in man. Quart J Exp Physiol 1957; 42:303-310.

4. Marino PL, Lamb TW. Effects of CO_2 and extracellular H+ iontophoresis on single cell activity in the cat brainstem. J Appl Physiol 1975; 38:688-695.

5. Forster RE II, DuBois AB, Briscoe WA, Fisher AB. The Lung: Physiological Basis of Pulmonary Function Tests. 3rd ed. Chicago: Year Book Medical Publishers, 1986:235-247.

6. Brahm J. The red cell anion-transport system: kinetics and physiologic implications. In Gunn RB, Parker C (eds). Cell Physiology of Blood. New York: Rockefeller Press, 1988; 142-150.

7. Katz AM. Ernest Henry Starling, his predecessors, and the 'Law of the Heart'. Circulation 2002; 106:2986-2992.

8. Guyton AG, Jones CE, Coleman TG. Peripheral vascular contribution to cardiac output regulation – the concept of "venous return". In: Circulatory Physiology: Cardiac Output and its Regulation. Philadelphia: W.B. Saunders, 1973:173-187.

9. Little RC, Little WC. Physiology of the Heart and Circulation. 2nd ed., Chicago: Yearbook Medical Publishers, 1989: pp. 47 and 229.

10. Pothier R. Astronauts beat air crisis by do-it-yourself gadget. Detroit Free Press, April 16, 1970.

Is O_2 transport the principal function of hemoglobin?

2

"When we all think alike, then no one is thinking."

Walter Lipmann, 1915

All but one of the vertebrate species employ hemoglobin as a transport vehicle for oxygen, the exception being Antarctic ice-fishes, whose diaphanous blood is devoid of hemoglobin and red blood cells (1). The perception that hemoglobin is all about O_2 delivery is, however, a myopic view, because it considers only the supply side of metabolism. The first chapter demonstrated that the cardiorespiratory system is more concerned with eliminating a metabolic waste product (CO_2) than delivering O_2 to tissues. This chapter will show that this also applies to the hemoglobin-red blood cell unit (also known as the *erythron*), and in the process of doing this, some features of hemoglobin and red blood cells will be presented that may have escaped your attention.

THE BURDEN OF THE ERYTHRON

One feature of the hemoglobin-red blood cell unit (the erythron) that receives little attention is its massive size, and the associated burden of manufacturing, maintaining, and moving a mass of this size (see Table 2.1). This is relevant because the burden imposed by the size of the erythron is not an intelligent design for an energy-supply process like O_2 delivery (which should be carried out at a limited energy cost). The implications of this are addressed later in the chapter.

Abundance of Hemoglobin

The concentration of hemoglobin is traditionally expressed in grams per deciliter (g/100 mL) rather than grams per liter (g/L), and this creates the tendency to underestimate the size of the hemoglobin pool. A representative hemoglobin concentration for a healthy adult is 15 g/dL, which is 150 grams per liter of blood. For a normal blood volume of 5 liters, the total mass of hemoglobin will be 750 grams (1.65 lbs). In comparison, the pump that propels this 750 grams through the circulatory system (i.e., the heart) has a mass of only 300 grams (0.6 lbs). This is a significant mismatch (think of a 170 lb individual who must move an object that weighs 425 lbs), but things get much worse with the addition of the red cell mass.

TABLE 2.1	Tally Sheet for the Erythron[†]
Hemoglobin	• Concentration: 150 grams per liter • Total Mass: 750 grams[*]
Red Blood Cells	• Concentration: 5.4 trillion cells per liter • Total Number: 27 trillion cells[*] • Replacement Rate: 1% (275 billion cells) daily • Red Cell Mass: 2 liters or 2 kilograms
Erythron	• Total Mass: 2.75 kilograms

[†]Values shown are representative values for healthy adults.
[*]Pertains to a blood volume of 5 liters.

Abundance of Red Blood Cells

Hemoglobin cannot roam free in plasma because it is broken down within a few hours, and the heme groups that are released are capable of damaging the vascular endothelium (an oxidative injury attributed to the iron in heme) (2). In addition, oxyhemoglobin is a scavenger of nitric oxide (3), and this promotes vasoconstriction, vascular thrombosis, and impaired blood flow. These adverse effects create a teleological need for an enclosure like red blood cells (RBCs) to sequester hemoglobin and prevent circulatory damage. (The "red blood cell" appellation is actually a misnomer, because RBCs lack a nucleus and have no mitochondria, and thus cannot be classified as eukaryotic cells. The term "red blood corpuscle" is more appropriate, but has not gained acceptance.) Unfortunately, the presence of RBCs creates its own circulatory problems, as described later.

The number of circulating RBCs is astonishing: i.e., each liter of blood contains an average of 5.4 trillion (5.4×10^{12}) RBCs in adult males (with about 12% fewer RBCs in adult females) (4). At a normal blood volume of 5 liters, there is a total of *27 trillion RBCs in the blood*. To place this number in perspective, the total number of cells in the human body is estimated at 37 trillion (5), which means the number of circulating RBCs represents almost 75% of all the cells in the human body! About 1% of circulating RBCs must be replaced daily (6), and this requires the production of (0.01 x 27.5 trillion) 275 billion RBCs every 24 hours, or 190 million RBCs every minute. And don't forget that every RBC contains about 300 million hemoglobin molecules that must be replaced. The energy cost of this task is not reported, but is unlikely to be inconsequential.

Mass of the Erythron

The normal red cell mass is about 2 L or 2 kg (5), and if this is combined with the normal mass of Hb derived earlier (i.e., 750 grams), the total mass of the erythron is 2.75 kg. This represents about 4% of body weight (for a 70 kg adult), and is greater than the mass of the liver (1.5 kg), brain (1.4 kg), lungs (1 kg), heart (0.3 kg), and kidneys (0.3 kg each) (7). In fact, *the erythron mass is larger than all the internal organs in the body except skeletal muscle.*

The heart has the burden of moving the erythron mass, and Figure 2.1 provides a visual image of the mismatch in size between the erythron and the heart. The erythron is 9 times heavier than the heart, and the work involved in moving such a mass helps to explain why the heart has the highest weight-adjusted O$_2$ consumption (94 mL/min/kg) of any organ in the body (7).

The burden imposed by the mass of the erythron is demonstrated by Newton's Second Law of Motion, which states that the force needed to set a body in motion (or change its motion) is directly related to the mass of the body and its acceleration (8): i.e.,

$$\text{Force} = \text{mass} \times \text{acceleration} \tag{2.1}$$

The larger the mass, the greater the force needed to propel it. (The force in this case is the driving pressure for blood flow, which is created by the strength of cardiac contractions.) This force must also overcome any resistive forces that oppose movement. Friction is the opposing force for the movement of solid objects along a surface, while the opposing force for the flow of fluids is the *viscosity* of the fluid (which has been described as the "gooiness" of a fluid). Blood viscosity then adds to the burden of moving the erythron mass.

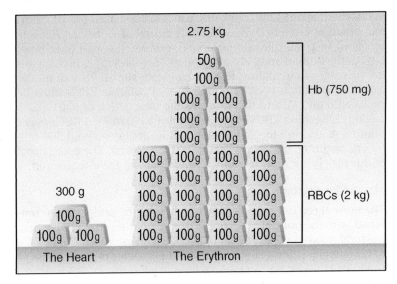

FIGURE 2.1 Visual representation of the mismatch between the mass of the erythron (hemoglobin and red blood cells) and the mass of the pump (the heart) that is burdened with moving the erythron through the circulatory system. Individual units represent weighted bars that each weigh 100 grams.

Blood Viscosity

The principal determinant of blood viscosity is the density or concentration of RBCs (i.e., the hematocrit), while abnormalities in the deformability and aggregation of RBCs add to the viscosity effect (9). Plasma is about 1.8 times more viscous than water, primarily because of its protein content, but plasma viscosity contributes little to the viscosity of whole blood. The flow impediment created by blood viscosity is described in Chapter 6, but the following observation is instructive. For flow through rigid tubes with a diameter of 100µ (the typical diameter of resistance vessels in the body) the flow rate of a cell-free hemoglobin solution is 30% greater than the flow rate of an RBC-containing fluid with the same amount of hemoglobin (10).

Summary

The burden created by the erythron includes the following:

1. The metabolic cost of producing and maintaining a mass that

is greater than all the internal organs of the body except skeletal muscle.

2. The cardiac work needed to circulate this mass, and to overcome the resistance created by the viscosity effects of RBCs.

The energy cost of this burden is excessive for an energy-supply process like O_2 delivery. Since the human body appears to operate by intelligent design (my bias), then the erythron should be doing more than delivering O_2 to tissues, to justify its excessive cost. Indirect evidence of this is presented next.

The Erythron and O_2 Delivery

Evidence that the erythron is not solely dedicated to O_2 delivery is provided in Figure 2.2. This graph shows the relationship between systemic O_2 delivery (DO_2) and O_2 uptake into tissues (VO_2). (*Note:* since O_2 is not stored in tissues, the O_2 uptake into tissues is equivalent to the O_2 consumption.) The boxes above both points on the graph show the O_2 saturation of hemoglobin in arterial and venous blood (SaO_2 and SvO_2, respectively). The $SaO_2 - SvO_2$ difference expresses the fraction of the hemoglobin molecules that have desaturated and released O_2 into the tissues.

In the box above the "normal" point, the ($SaO_2 - SvO_2$) difference is 0.23 (23%), indicating that about one-quarter of the hemoglobin molecules have desaturated and released O_2 into the tissues, and the SvO_2 is 0.75, indicating that 75% of the hemoglobin molecules in venous blood remain fully saturated with oxygen. Thus, three-quarters of the circulating hemoglobin molecules do not release O_2 into the tissues under normal conditions.

As the DO_2 is decreased from the normal point (e.g., by decreasing cardiac output), the VO_2 initially remains unchanged. This is possible because of an increase in O_2 extraction from hemoglobin, which is reflected by an increase in the $SaO_2 - SvO_2$ difference. This relationship is stated below:

$$VO_2 = DO_2 \times (SaO_2 - SvO_2) \qquad (2.2)$$

As the DO_2 continues to decrease, the increase in O_2 extraction has a limit, which is shown as the point of maximal O_2 extraction in Figure 2.2. At this point, the ($SaO_2 - SvO_2$) difference has increased to 0.48 (indicating that 50% of the hemoglobin molecules have desaturated and released their O_2 into the tissues), while the SvO_2 has decreased to 0.50 (indicating that 50% of the hemoglo-

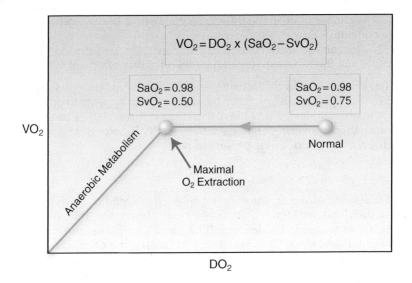

FIGURE 2.2 Graph of the relationship between systemic O_2 delivery (DO_2) and O_2 uptake (VO_2). SaO_2 and SvO_2 represent the O_2 saturation of hemoglobin in arterial and venous blood, respectively. The ($SaO_2 - SvO_2$) difference is the extent of O_2 desaturation in capillary blood. See text for further explanation.

bin molecules remain fully saturated with O_2). Further decreases in DO_2 beyond this point will result in proportional decreases in VO_2 and the onset of anaerobic metabolism. Since the maximum O_2 extraction is 50%, this means that half of the hemoglobin molecules never release O_2 into the tissues, even when tissue oxygenation is impaired. This is evidence that the erythron mass is much larger than needed for O_2 delivery, which supports the notion mentioned earlier that the erythron is involved with more than O_2 delivery. (The erythron also transports CO_2, which is described later in the chapter.)

Exercise

The condition described for Figure 2.2 is based on a primary decrease in O_2 delivery (i.e., from anemia, hypoxia, or a decrease in cardiac output), and this differs from a condition like exercise, where there is a primary increase in VO_2. In the latter condition, the increase in O_2 consumption could increase the gradient for O_2 movement into tissues, thereby increasing the O_2 extraction from hemoglobin. The maximum O_2 extraction can increase to 70–75% during strenuous exercise, in fit athletes. However, this leaves a considerable fraction ($\geq 25\%$) of the hemoglobin pool that never-releases O_2 into the tissues. (This amounts to at least 25% of 2.5 kg, or 625 mg of excess hemoglobin and RBCs, which is more than twice the mass of the heart.)

A Novel View of the Erythron

The reluctance of hemoglobin to release O_2 into the tissues is contrary to the popular perception that hemoglobin is all about delivering O_2 to the tissues. In fact, hemoglobin is releasing only what is needed to support aerobic metabolism. This view of the erythron as a "holding tank" for O_2 is supported by the fact that 98% of all the O_2 in the body is bound to hemoglobin (see Table 3.1). By limiting the release of O_2 into the tissues, the erythron is also limiting the risk of oxygen-related cell injury, which is a form of antioxidant protection. Thus, *a molecule that is billed as promoting tissue oxygenation is actually restricting tissue oxygenation*, to protect the tissues from the damaging effects of oxygen.

CARBON DIOXIDE TRANSPORT

Carbon dioxide is the principal end-product of metabolism, and must be transported to the lungs for elimination. The transport of CO_2 in blood was introduced in Chapter 1, and is presented in more detail here, with a focus on the important role of the erythron in CO_2 transport.

Transport Scheme

The centerpiece of CO_2 transport is the reaction of CO_2 with water, which produces carbonic acid (H_2CO_3), a weak acid that immediately dissociates into hydrogen ions (H^+) and bicarbonate ions ($HCO3^-$). This reaction is shown below:

$$CO_2 + H_2O \rightarrow H_2CO_3 \rightarrow H^+ + HCO_3^- \qquad (2.3)$$

As mentioned in Chapter 1, the participation of CO_2 in this reaction allows aqueous fluids to hold large volumes of CO_2 (because the chemical reaction removes CO_2, thereby maintaining a gradient that draws CO_2 into solution). In fact, the volume of CO_2 can exceed the volume of the fluid if the CO_2 pressure is sufficiently elevated. This explains why there is an estimated 130 liters of CO_2 in the human body (11), while the average-sized adult has only 40–50 liters of total body water.

Carbon dioxide is transported as the products of carbonic acid dissociation (H^+ and HCO_3^-), and the transport scheme is shown in Figure 2.3. Dissolved CO_2 accounts for only 5% of CO_2 transport (12), and is not included in the figure. The CO_2 hydration reaction is sluggish, and the reaction time (40 seconds) is too slow to reach completion before venous blood reaches the lungs. However, in the presence of the enzyme *carbonic anhydrase*, the reaction time is less than 10 milliseconds (11). Carbonic anhydrase is located in RBCs but not in plasma, so the principal site of carbonic acid production is in RBCs. The hydrogen ions that are generated are buffered by the histidine molecules in hemoglobin, while the bicarbonate ions are pumped back into the plasma in exchange for chloride ions (for electrical neutrality) (12). Because the dissociation products of carbonic acid do not accumulate in RBCs, the CO_2 hydration reaction will continue unabated, as long as there is available substrate (CO_2). This creates a "sink" for CO_2 transport in RBCs.

Hemoglobin as a Buffer

Hemoglobin is the principal vehicle for CO_2 transport by virtue of its ability to absorb the H^+ produced by the dissociation of carbonic acid. The actions of hemoglobin as a buffer were discovered in the 1930s, but this aspect of hemoglobin function is rarely recognized in modern medicine. The buffering capacity of hemoglobin is attributed to its 38 histidine molecules, and more specifically, to the imidazole ring in the histidine molecule. (Imidazole is a 5-member ring made up of carbon and nitrogen atoms, and can function as an acid or a base.) Histidine is the only amino acid that acts as a buffer in the physiological pH range. It is most effective as a buffer in the pH range of 6–8 (12), whereas the carbonic acid-bicarbonate buffer system is most effective in the pH range of 5–7 (13). This means that *hemoglobin is a more effective buffer than bicarbonate in the physiological pH range* (7.0–7.6).

The buffering capacity of hemoglobin is compared to the plasma proteins in Table 2.2 (13). The inherent buffer capacity of hemoglobin is about 50% higher than plasma proteins, but as a result of the much higher concentration of hemoglobin, the total buffering capacity of hemoglobin is 6 times greater than the plasma proteins. This shows the importance of the large size of the hemoglobin pool for the transport of CO_2.

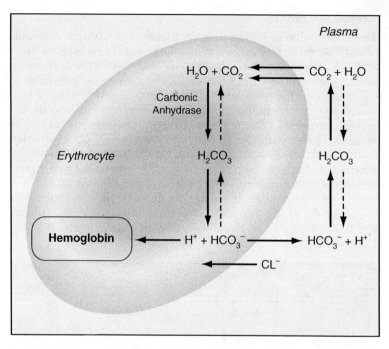

FIGURE 2.3 Chemical reactions involved in the transport of CO_2 in blood. Solid arrows indicate the favored direction of each reaction. See text for further explanation.

Table 2.2	Buffering Capacity of Blood Proteins	
	Hemoglobin	**Plasma Proteins**
Inherent Buffer Capacity	0.18 mEq H⁺/g	0.11 mEq H⁺/g
Concentration in Whole Blood	150 g/L	38.5 g/L
Total Buffer Capacity	27.5 mEq H⁺/L	4.24 mEq H⁺/L

From Reference 13.

The Haldane Effect

The information in Table 2.3 shows that the CO_2 content in venous blood is 40 mL/L higher than in arterial blood. There is also a higher PCO_2 in venous blood, but this is responsible for only about half of the increment in CO_2 content. The remaining increment in CO_2 content is the result of O_2 desaturation of hemoglobin, which increases both the buffering capacity of hemoglobin, and the reactions between CO_2 and amino groups in hemoglobin (12). The increased affinity for CO_2 in deoxygenated hemoglobin is known as the "Haldane Effect"(discovered by the Scottish physiologist, John Scott Haldane), and it facilitates the venous transport (and subsequent elimination) of CO_2. It is especially relevant in the setting of hypermetabolism: i.e., an increase in metabolic rate increases the O_2 desaturation of hemoglobin in capillary blood, and this not only delivers more O_2 into the tissues, it also helps to transport the extra CO_2 that is produced.

Table 2.3	Hemoglobin-bound O_2 and CO_2 in Blood		
	Arterial Blood	**Venous Blood**	**Total**
Blood Volume	1.25 L	3.75 L	5.0 L
Oxygen			
HbO_2/Total Hb	0.98	0.75	—
HbO_2 Content[1]	197 mL/L	151 mL/L	—
HbO_2 Volume	246 mL	566 mL	812 mL
Carbon Dioxide			
PCO_2 (mm Hg)	40	46	—
$HbCO_2$ Content[2]	466 mL/L	504 mL/L	—
$HbCO_2$ Volume	583 mL	1,890 mL	2,473 mL

[1]Based on calculations shown in Chapter 3.
[2]From Reference 12.

Why O_2 Transport is Not the Principal Function of Hemoglobin

Hemoglobin is the principal transport vehicle for both O_2 and CO_2, and accounts for 98% of O_2 transport (see Chapter 3), and 95% of

CO_2 transport (12). The information in Table 2.3 is a comparison of the hemoglobin-bound O_2 and hemoglobin-bound CO_2 in both arterial and venous blood. (The hemoglobin-bound CO_2 represents the binding of CO_2 as H^+.) Note that *the volume of CO_2 transported by hemoglobin is about three times greater than the volume of O_2 transported.* This explains why the erythron mass is much larger than needed for O_2 transport, and it also answers the question posed in the title of this chapter, because it indicates that the *principal function of hemoglobin is the transport of CO_2, not O_2.* End of story.

Primacy of CO_2 Removal Over O_2 Delivery

Oxygen delivery to the tissues is widely regarded as the principal concern of the heart, lungs, and hemoglobin-containing RBCs (the erythron). However, the first chapter demonstrated that the ventilatory effort is controlled by CO_2, not O_2, and that cardiac output influences CO_2 transport more than O_2 transport, while this chapter shows that the erythron is more involved with the transport of CO_2 rather than O_2. Taken together, this seems to indicate that the systems presumed to be dedicated to O_2 delivery are actually more concerned with CO_2 removal.

The perceived importance of O_2 delivery is addressed from a different angle in the next chapter, which shows that the tissues normally operate in an oxygen-poor environment.

SUMMATION

The combined mass of hemoglobin and RBCs (the erythron) is larger than any internal organ in the body except skeletal muscle. However, 25–50% of this mass never releases O_2 into the tissues, even when tissue oxygenation is impaired.

The erythron mass is much larger than needed for O_2 transport because it also transports CO_2 (as H^+) in a volume that is 3 times greater than the volume of O_2 transported. The larger transport volume of CO_2 indicates that the principal function of hemoglobin is the transport of CO_2, not O_2.

REFERENCES

1. Sidell BD, O'Brien KM. When bad things happen to good fish: the loss of hemoglobin and myoglobin expression in Antarctic icefishes. J Exp Biol 2006; 209:1791-1802.
2. Belcher JD, Beckman JD, Balla G, et al. Heme degradation and vascular injury. Antiox Redox Sign 2010; 12:233-248.

3. Schechter AN, Gladwin MT. Hemoglobin and the paracrine and endocrine functions of nitric oxide. N Engl J Med 2003; 348:1483-1485.

4. Walker RH, ed. American Association of Blood Banks Technical Manual. 10th ed. Arlington, VA: American Association of Blood Banks, 1990:649

5. Bianconi E, Piovesan A, Facchin F, et al. An estimation of the number of cells in the human body. Ann Human Biol 2013; 40:463-471.

6. Hillman RS, Finch CA. Red Cell Manual. 6th ed. Philadelphia: F.A. Davis, Co., 1992:33.

7. Diem K, Lentner C, eds. Documenta Geigy Scientific Tables. 7th ed. Basel: Geigy, 1970:539.

8. Arianrhod R. Einstein's Heroes: Imagining the world through the language of mathematics. Oxford: Oxford University Press, 2005:42-50.

9. Baskurt OK, Meiselman HJ. Blood rheology and hemodynamics. Semin Thromb Hemost 2003; 29:435-450.

10. Charm SE, Kurland GS. Blood Flow and Microcirculation. New York: John Wiley & Sons, 1974:158-159.

11. Henneberg S, Soderberg D, Groth T, et al. Carbon dioxide production during mechanical ventilation. Crit Care Med 1987; 15:8-13.

12. Nunn JF. Carriage of carbon dioxide in blood. In: Nunn's Applied Respiratory Physiology, 4th ed. Oxford: Butterworth-Heinemann, 1993:219-229.

13. Comroe JH Jr. Physiology of respiration. 2nd ed. Chicago, Yearbook Med Publishers, 1974:201-210.

3

How much oxygen is in tissues?

"The simplest protection against oxygen toxicity is to hide."

Nick Lane (*a*)

We all know that hemoglobin is needed to transport oxygen to the tissues because oxygen does not readily dissolve in aqueous fluids like plasma. However, once oxygen is released from hemoglobin and enters the tissues, the only available oxygen is the small amount that is dissolved in the intracellular and extracellular fluids. This chapter documents the paucity of oxygen in tissues, and especially in cells, and shows how aerobic metabolism can operate in such an oxygen-poor environment. The intention here is to show that the cells don't need a lot of oxygen to function normally, and to point out that the low-oxygen environment in tissues is advantageous because it allows our vital cell components to "hide" from the damaging effects of oxygen (which are described in the second section of the book).

OXYGEN PRESSURES

The Oxygen Cascade

The movement of O_2 along the route from the lungs to the interior of cells is associated with a steady and precipitous decline in the partial pressure of O_2 (PO_2). This "oxygen cascade" is illustrated in Figure 3.1, which shows typical PO_2 values at major points along the oxygen transport route, from ambient air (at sea level) to the interior of cells. The large, initial drop in PO_2 from atmospheric air to alveolar gas is a dilutional effect created by the humidification of inhaled air and by the CO_2 that enters the alveoli from venous blood. This is followed by a small drop in PO_2 from alveolar gas to pulmonary capillary blood, which is attributed to venous blood from the upper airways that drains into the pulmonary veins and bypasses the pulmonary capillaries. (This *alveolar-arterial PO_2 gradient* is increased by any condition that impairs gas exchange in the lungs.) Following this, there is a considerable drop in PO_2 from arterial blood to blood in the systemic capillaries. This is mainly due to the movement of O_2 out of the capillaries and into the tissues, but there is also evidence of a longitudinal PO_2 gradient along the arterial network (attributed to O_2 consumption in the walls of arteries, and to the movement of O_2 out of arterioles and into the tissues) (1).

The final stages of O_2 transport involve the movement of O_2 from capillary blood into the tissues, where O_2 moves through the interstitial fluid, and enters cells, to reach its final destination in mitochondria. There is a substantial drop in PO_2 along this route, resulting in an intracellular PO_2 that is ≤ 5 mm Hg (see later).

Tissue PO_2

Direct measurements of tissue PO_2 are not routinely available in clinical practice. Near-infrared spectroscopy is available as a non-invasive method for monitoring the O_2 saturation of hemoglobin in the systemic microcirculation (mostly in small venules) (2). However, this measure (i.e., the venous O_2 saturation) is a reflection of the balance between O_2 delivery and O_2 consumption, and has no direct correlation with tissue PO_2. The bulk of tissue PO_2 measurements are from animal studies, and a brief description of the methodology is warranted.

Methodology

The traditional method for measuring the PO_2 in biological fluids is the oxygen-sensitive polarographic electrode, introduced in the early 1960s by Leland Clark Jr. (3). The "Clark electrode" has a platinum cathode that is in contact with the fluid sample. A small polarizing voltage is applied to the cathode to induce the electrolytic reduction of O_2 to H_2O in the fluid, and the resulting transfer of electrons to the cathode produces a current that is proportional to the PO_2 in the fluid. Clark electrodes are used to measure the PO_2 in blood samples, and they have been miniaturized for the measurement of PO_2 in tissues and in cells (4). Tissue penetration by these electrodes can disrupt cells and small blood vessels, which is a source of spurious measurements.

The risk of tissue disruption with Clark electrodes is eliminated by the more recently introduced optical method of O_2 detection, which is noninvasive. Optical electrodes or "optodes" emit light waves that excite O_2-sensitive luminescent dyes. The subsequent phosphorescence is quenched by O_2, and the decay rate of the phosphorescence is inversely proportional to the PO_2 in the surrounding fluid (5). Optodes have largely replaced polarographic

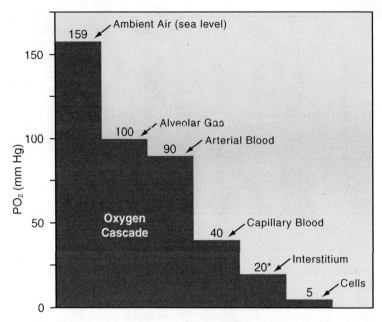

FIGURE 3.1 Illustration of the cascading decline in PO_2 that occurs as oxygen moves from atmospheric air to parenchymal cells in tissues. The asterisk indicates that interstitial PO_2 can vary in individual organs. See text for further details.

electrodes for tissue PO_2 recordings, but these electrodes can produce spuriously high measurements if the recording site is adjacent to a blood vessel.

Measurements

Tissue PO_2 recordings are considered a reflection of the average PO_2 in interstitial fluid, and they typically involve multiple recordings at different recording sites. The result is a frequency histogram like the one shown in Figure 3.2 (6), which provides a PO_2 profile for the field of study. The histogram in this case has a Gaussian or "normal" distribution, indicating that mean PO_2 (19.6 mm Hg) is a valid representation of the average PO_2 in the surrounding interstitial fluid.

The tissue PO_2 can vary in different organs, and in different regions of the same organ. Examples of tissue PO_2 measurements in different organs (from animal studies) is shown in Table 3.1 (6-11).

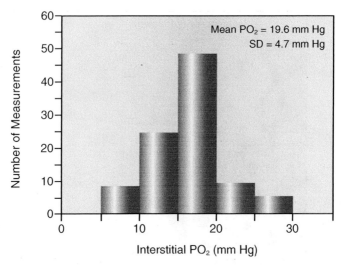

FIGURE 3.2 Frequency histogram of tissue (interstitial) PO_2 measurements from an *in situ* skeletal muscle preparation that allowed microscopic visualization of the underlying tissue. Individual measurements were taken from different points along a recording grid. From data in Reference 6.

Note that the tissue PO_2 is remarkably similar (20–25 mm Hg) in four of the six organs, while the lens of the eye is almost devoid of oxygen. The lack of O_2 in the lens has a protective effect, because the oxidation of lens proteins is the principal source of cataract formation (11). The link between O_2 and cataracts is supported by reports of accelerated cataract formation following hyperbaric oxygen therapy (12).

Intracellular PO_2

Direct measurements of intracellular PO_2 are not abundant, but the available studies show that there is an oxygen-poor environment in cells. In one study of resting skeletal muscle cells (studied *in situ*), the intracellular PO_2 was 5.4 ± 0.5 mm Hg (mean$\pm$SD), and 70 of the 184 cells tested (38%) had an intracellular $PO_2 < 1$ mm Hg (13). Another study of *in situ* skeletal muscle found that the intracellular PO_2 fell to 1.4 mm Hg when the muscle was stimulated to 95% of its maximum O_2 consumption (14). Finally, in studies of isolated cardiac myocytes, the intracellular PO_2 was 0.2–2.4 mm Hg (14).

Table 3.1   Tissue PO$_2$ Recordings in Various Tissues

Tissue	Mean PO$_2$ (mm Hg)	Reference #
Cerebral Cortex	24.5	7
Liver	23.4	8
Myocardium	19.7	9
Skeletal Muscle	19.6	6
Bone Marrow	13.3	10
Ocular Lens	1.6	11

Critical PO$_2$

The ability to conduct aerobic metabolism in a low-oxygen environment is explained by observations of the "critical PO$_2$," which is defined as the intracellular PO$_2$ at which O$_2$ consumption (or ATP production) begins to decline. Animal studies have reported a critical PO$_2 \leq 0.5$ mm Hg in cardiac and skeletal muscle (14, 15), and 0.92–1.54 mm Hg in isolated renal mitochondria (16). These numbers indicate that aerobic metabolism can run on "fumes" of oxygen.

TOTAL BODY OXYGEN

The PO$_2$ measurement provides little information about the amount of available oxygen at a particular site. Since oxygen needs are defined by the oxygen consumption, which is expressed in mL/min, the volume of oxygen (in mLs) is the best measure of oxygenation. Estimates of the oxygen volumes in Table 3.2 show how much oxygen is in the body of an average-sized adult, and how it is distributed. Note that there is less than one liter of oxygen in the body, and that almost all of it (98%) is bound to hemoglobin, leaving very little oxygen in the tissues. The oxygen volume estimates in this table are the centerpiece of the chapter, and thus a description of how they are derived seems warranted.

Table 3.2   Distribution of Total Body Oxygen

Component	Volume	O_2 Concentration	Volume of O_2
Hemoglobin-Bound O_2			
Arterial Blood	1.25 L	197 mL/L	246 mL (30%)
Venous Blood	3.75 L	151 mL/L	566 mL (70%)
	Total: 5.0 L		Total: 812 mL
Plasma O_2			
Plasma (arterial)	0.7 L	2.9 mL/L	2.0 mL
Plasma (venous)	2.1 L	1.2 mL/L	2.5 mL
	Total: 2.8 L		Total: 4.5 mL
Tissue O_2			
Interstitial Fluid	14 L	0.75 mL/L	10.5 mL
Parenchymal Cells	23 L	0.15 mL/L	3.5 mL
			Total: 14.0 mL

Total O_2 in Blood

The total volume of oxygen in blood is dependent on the concentration of hemoglobin-bound O_2 and plasma O_2 in arterial and venous blood, as well as the arterial and venous blood volumes.

Hemoglobin-Bound O_2

The concentration of hemoglobin-bound O_2 (HbO_2) is described by the following equation:

$$HbO_2 = 1.34 \times [Hb] \times SO_2 \ (mL/L) \qquad (3.1)$$

where [Hb] is the hemoglobin concentration (in g/L), 1.34 is the O_2 carrying capacity of hemoglobin (in mL/g), and SO_2 is the O_2 saturation of hemoglobin (expressed as the ratio of oxygenated hemoglobin to total hemoglobin). This equation states that each gram of hemoglobin will bind 1.34 mL O_2 when it is fully saturated with O_2 (i.e., when $SO_2 = 1.0$).

The HbO_2 in arterial blood is determined using a [Hb] of 150 g/L (equivalent to 15 g/dL) and an arterial SO_2 (SaO_2) of 0.98:

$$HbO_2(a) = 1.34 \times 150 \times 0.98 = 197 \text{ mL/L} \qquad (3.2)$$

The HbO_2 in venous blood is determined using the same [Hb] of 150 g/L and a venous SO_2 (SvO_2) of 0.75:

$$HbO_2(v) = 1.34 \times 150 \times 0.75 = 151 \text{ mL/L} \qquad (3.3)$$

The volume of HbO_2 in arterial and venous blood is calculated using a blood volume of 5 liters, with 75% of the blood volume (3.75 L) in the veins, and 25% (1.25 L) in the arteries.

$$\text{Volume of } HbO_2(a) = 197 \times 1.25 = 246 \text{ mL} \qquad (3.4)$$

$$\text{Volume of } HbO_2(v) = 151 \times 3.75 = 566 \text{ mL} \qquad (3.5)$$

The total volume of HbO_2 is 812 mL. Note that the volume of HbO_2 in venous blood is more than double the volume in arterial blood, and that *venous blood contains 70% of the hemoglobin-bound O_2 in the blood* (see Table 3.2). This indicates that a large fraction of hemoglobin-bound O_2 is withheld from the tissues under normal conditions, which supports the proposal in Chapter 2 that hemoglobin helps to limit or restrict tissue oxygenation.

Dissolved O_2

The oxygen that is not bound to hemoglobin is physically dissolved in body fluids. The concentration of dissolved O_2 is determined using *Henry's Law* (discovered by William Henry, a 19th century British chemist), which states that the concentration of a dissolved gas in aqueous fluids is proportional to the pressure of the gas above the fluid, with a proportionality factor that varies inversely with the temperature of the fluid (17). This is expressed below for the concentration of dissolved O_2:

$$\text{Dissolved } O_2 = \alpha \times PO_2 \qquad (3.6)$$

α is the proportionality factor, also known as the solubility coefficient. At 37°C, the solubility coefficient for oxygen in plasma is 0.03 mL/L/mmHg (18), which means that at a PO_2 of 100 mm Hg, only 3 mL of O_2 will dissolve in each liter of plasma. This indicates that *oxygen does not readily dissolve in aqueous fluids*.

The O_2 concentration in plasma is separated into arterial and venous components, similar to the hemoglobin-bound O_2. The arterial component is determined using an arterial PO_2 of 98 mm Hg, while a PO_2 of 40 mm Hg is used for the venous component:

$$\text{Plasma } O_2(a) = 0.03 \times 98 = 2.9 \text{ mL/L} \qquad (3.7)$$

$$\text{Plasma } O_2(v) = 0.03 \times 40 = 1.2 \text{ mL/L} \qquad (3.8)$$

To calculate the volume of dissolved O_2 in plasma, it is necessary to determine the plasma volume. At a hematocrit of 45%, the plasma volume should be 55% of the blood volume, so the arterial plasma volume will be 0.55×1.25 L = 0.7 L, and the venous plasma volume will be 0.55×3.75 L = 2.1 L. The volume of dissolved O_2 in arterial and venous plasma is then:

$$\text{Volume of Plasma } O_2(a) = 0.7 \times 2.9 = 2.0 \text{ mL} \qquad (3.9)$$

$$\text{Volume of Plasma } O_2(v) = 2.1 \times 1.2 = 2.5 \text{ mL} \qquad (3.10)$$

Comparing the volume of dissolved O_2 in plasma (4.5 mL), with the volume of Hb-bound O_2 (812 mL) shows that *only 0.6% of the oxygen in blood is dissolved in plasma*. Because oxygen does not readily dissolve in plasma, the plasma can serve as an impediment to the movement of oxygen from RBCs into the tissues (19).

Total O_2 in Tissues

We finally address the question in the title of the chapter: i.e., how much oxygen is in the tissues of the body? Since only the dissolved fraction of O_2 is in tissues, not much is expected.

Interstitial O_2

The concentration of O_2 in interstitial fluid is determined with equation 3.6, using the solubility coefficient for plasma (i.e., aqueous fluids) and a PO_2 of 25 mm Hg (which is the highest tissue PO_2 in Table 3.1).

$$\text{Interstitial } O_2 = 0.03 \times 25 = 0.75 \text{ ml/L} \qquad (3.11)$$

The volume of interstitial fluid is determined using the following assumptions (20): 1) Total body water (TBW) is 60% of the lean body weight. 2) Extracellular volume (ECV) represents 40% of the TBW, and 3) the interstitial volume is equivalent to the ECV minus the plasma volume. For a 70 kg adult, the TBW will be $0.6 \times 70 = 42$ liters, ECV will be $0.4 \times 42 = 16.8$ liters, and the interstitial volume will be $16.8 - 2.8 = 14$ liters. Therefore:

$$\text{Volume of Interstitial Fluid } O_2 = 0.75 \times 14 \text{ L} = 10.5 \text{ mL} \qquad (3.12)$$

That's not much O_2, and there's even less in cells.

Intracellular O_2

The O_2 concentration in cells is determined using an intracellular PO_2 of 5 mm Hg, which is a generous value based on the studies mentioned previously.

$$\text{Intracellular } O_2 = 0.03 \times 5 = 0.15 \text{ mL/L} \qquad (3.13)$$

The volume of O_2 in cells pertains only to parenchymal cells (as distinguished from blood cells). The volume of parenchymal cells is determined using the following assumptions: 1) the TBW is 60% of lean body weight, 2) the intracellular volume (ICV) is 60% of the TBW, and 3) the parenchymal cell volume is the ICV minus the red cell volume (which is 45% of the blood volume). For a 70 kg adult with a blood volume of 5 liters, the TBW is 42 liters, the ICV is 0.6 x 42 = 25.2 liters, the red cell volume is 0.45 x 5 = 2.3 liters, and the parenchymal cell volume is 25.2 – 2.3 = 22.9 (rounded to 23) liters. Therefore:

$$\text{Volume of Intracellular } O_2 = 0.15 \times 23 \text{ L} = 3.5 \text{ mL} \qquad (3.14)$$

Thus, the total volume of O_2 in the parenchymal cells of the body is equivalent to less than one teaspoonful of liquid.

Our Oxygen-Poor Tissues

The question in the title of the chapter can now be answered: i.e, *in the average-sized adult, the total volume of oxygen in tissues (interstitium plus cells) is equivalent to about one tablespoonful of liquid (14 mL), and less than one teaspoonful (3.5 mL) is located in cells.* This oxygen-poor environment is the result of the poor solubility of O_2 in aqueous fluids, and the reluctance of hemoglobin to release O_2 into the tissues (as described in Chapter 2). Aerobic metabolism can continue in such an environment because it is capable of running at extremely low oxygen levels (as shown by the "critical PO_2" data presented earlier).

Protective Effect of Water

The hydrophobic nature of oxygen allows water to serve as a protective shield against oxidation. This is easily demonstrated by the following exercise. Peel a potato and cut it into one-inch cubes. Leave half of the cubes exposed to air, and place the other half in a bowl of cold water. The potato cubes exposed to air will begin to turn brown after about 5–10 minutes (as a result of oxidation of polysaccharides in the potato), while the cubes submerged in cold water will not turn brown for hours. (You can also use an apple for this exercise, but the oxidation in air seems more pronounced with potatoes.)

As land creatures, we are constantly bathed in atmospheric oxygen, which creates a relentless threat of oxidative tissue injury. Fortunately, the adult human body is about 50–60% water by weight, and this water shields us from the damaging effects of atmospheric oxygen. The protective effect of water may explain why a fetus gestates in amniotic fluid, and why a microbe surrounds itself with an aqueous biofilm.

Countermeasures

Clinical interventions that are aimed at promoting tissue oxygenation are often met by countermeasures that prevent undesirable increases in oxygenation. Two examples of this are the vasoconstrictor response to oxygen inhalation (21), and the increase in blood viscosity from RBC transfusions (22). Both responses reduce blood flow, which limits the ability of these interventions to influence tissue oxygenation. (See Chapters 5 and 6 for more information on these responses.) These countermeasures are a testament to the importance of maintaining an oxygen-poor environment in tissues.

Man as a Microaerophile

Microaerophilic organisms require oxygen to survive, but they are also damaged by oxygen, and must live in an oxygen-poor environment. This description also seems to apply to the parenchymal cells of the human body. Therefore, although humans are considered to be "obligate aerobes" (i.e., organisms that require oxygen to survive, and exist in oxygen-rich environments), from the standpoint of our vital parts, we are more akin to microaerophilic organisms.

SUMMATION

Estimates of the total body oxygen in this chapter can be summarized as follows:

1. There is less than one liter of oxygen in the adult human body, and 98% of it is bound to hemoglobin, leaving very little oxygen (14 mL) in the tissues. The oxygen-poor environment in tissues is the result of the hydrophobic behavior of oxygen, and the reluctance of hemoglobin to release oxygen into the tissues.
2. The benefit of maintaining an oxygen-poor environment in tissues is the reduced risk of cell damage from oxidation.

Aerobic metabolism can continue in such an environment because it can run at PO_2 levels below 1 mm Hg.

3. Clinical interventions that promote tissue oxygenation often elicit countermeasures that protect tissues from undesirable increases in oxygenation. An example of this is the vasoconstrictor response to oxygen inhalation. Such countermeasures highlight the importance of maintaining a low-O_2 environment in our tissues.

REFERENCES

a. Lane, N, Oxygen: The Molecule that Made the World, Oxford: Oxford University Press, 2002; 196.

1. Keeley TP, Mann GE. Defining physiological normoxia for improved translation of cell physiology to animal models and humans. Physiol Rev 2019; 99:161-234.

2. Davies DJ, Su Z, Clancy MT, Lucas SJ, et al. Near-infrared spectroscopy in the monitoring of adult traumatic brain injury: a review. J Neurotrauma 2015; 32:933-941.

3. Severinghaus JW, Astrup, PB. History of blood gas analysis. IV. Leland Clark's oxygen electrode. J Clin Monit 1986; 2: 125–139.

4. Whalen WJ, Riley J, A microelectrode for measurement of intracellular PO_2. J Appl Physiol 1967; 23:798-801.

5. Papkovsky DB, Zhdanov AV. Phosphorescence based O_2 sensors – Essential tools for monitoring cell and tissue oxygenation and its impact on metabolism. Free Rad Biol Med 2016; 101:202-210.

6. Tsai AG, Johnson PC, Intaglietta M. Is the distribution of tissue pO_2 homogeneous? Antiox Redox Sign 2007; 9:979-984.

7. Smith R, Guilbeau E, Reneau D. The oxygen tension field within a discrete volume of cerebral cortex. Microvasc Res 1977; 13:233-240.

8. Jiang J, Nakashima T, Liu KJ, et al. Measurement of PO_2 in liver using EPR oximetry. J Appl Physiol 1996; 80:552-558.

9. Chacko SM, Khan M, Kuppusamy ML, et al. Myocardial oxygenation and functional recovery in infarct rat hearts transplanted with mesenchymal stem cells. Am J Physiol Heart Circ Physiol 2009; 296:H1263-H1273.

10. Spencer JA, Ferraro F, Roussakis E, et al. Direct measurement of local oxygen concentration in the bone marrow of live animals. Nature 2014; 508:269-273.

11. McNulty R, Wand H, Mathias R, et al. Regulation of tissue oxygen levels in the mammalian lens. J Physiol 2004; 559:883-898.

12. Palmquist B-M, Philipson B, Barr P-O. Nuclear cataract and myopia during hyperbaric oxygen therapy. Br J Ophthalmol 1984; 68:113-117.

13. Whalen WJ, Nair P. Intracellular PO_2 and its regulation in resting skeletal muscle of the guinea pig. Circ Res 1967; 21:251-261.

14. Gayeski EJ, Honig CR. Intracellular PO_2 in long axis of individual fibers in working dog gracilis muscle. Am J Physiol Heart Circ Physiol 1988; 254:H1179-H1186.

15. Wittenberg BA, Wittenberg JB. Oxygen pressure gradients in isolated cardiac myocytes. J Biol Chem 1985; 260:6548-6554.

16. Stolp W, Thiwman V, Weber D, Weiss Ch. Measurements of the critical PO_2 of renal mitochondria. Pflugers Arch 1971; 323:250-257.

17. Henry W. Experiments on the quantity of gases absorbed by water at different temperatures and under different pressures. Phil Trans R Soc Lond 1803; 93:29-274.

18. Christoforides C, Laasberg LH, Hedley-Whyte J. Effect of temperature on solubility of O_2 in human plasma. J Appl Physiol 1969; 26:56-60.

19. Hellums JD. The resistance to oxygen transport in the capillaries relative to that in the surrounding tissue. Microvasc Res 1977; 13:131-136.

20. Rose BD, Post TW. Clinical Physiology of Acid-Base and Electrolyte Disorders. 5th ed, New York: McGraw-Hill, 2001:682.

21. Farquhar H, Weatherall M, Wijesinghe M, et al. Systematic review of studies of the effects of hyperoxia on coronary blood flow. Am Heart J 2009; 158:371-377.

22. Baskrut OK, Meiselman HJ. Blood rheology and hemodynamics. Semin Thromb Hemost 2003; 29:435-450.

Is tissue hypoxia a common cause of death?

4

"If one were to name the universal factor in all death…
it would certainly be loss of oxygen."

Sherwin Nuland, MD (*a*)

One of the more pervasive beliefs about oxygen is stated (with uncompromising certainty) in the introductory quote, which identifies a lack of oxygen as the *sine qua non* for the death of aerobic organisms. This credo permeates all of clinical medicine and is especially evident in the management of acutely or seriously ill patients, where the primary concern is to promote the delivery of oxygen to tissues (e.g., with interventions like oxygen inhalation, mechanical ventilation, erythrocyte transfusions, and volume infusions to promote cardiac output). Yet there is no direct measure of tissue oxygenation to support any of this.

There are two sources for the perception that tissue hypoxia is the principal harbinger of cell death. (Tissue hypoxia is defined as tissue oxygenation that is inadequate for the needs of aerobic metabolism.) The first source is an inherent bias based on the necessity of oxygen for life as we know it. This creates the following type of flawed reasoning: "Since oxygen is necessary for life, then lack of oxygen must be necessary for death." The fallacy here is that oxygen is not the only factor necessary for life (other vital cell components are needed, such as DNA, proteins, cell membranes, etc.) and a defect in any of these other factors can be lethal. The second source comes from studies that show a direct correlation between clinical markers of tissue hypoxia and the likelihood of a fatal outcome in life-threatening conditions. The problem here is the unreliability of these clinical markers, as demonstrated in this chapter.

The notion that death is the result of an oxygen-poor environment is contrary to the information presented in Chapter 3, which demonstrated that an oxygen-poor environment is the normal state of affairs in our tissues. The information in this chapter will help to resolve this discrepancy.

LACTATE

The most widely used clinical marker of tissue hypoxia is an increase in the plasma lactate concentration, and this marker, far more than any other, has contributed to the perception that tissue hypoxia is a common cause of death.

The link between lactate production and tissue hypoxia can be traced back to the mid-19th century, when Louis Pasteur discovered that the fermentation of sugars by yeast was inhibited by aerating the yeast broth cultures (1). This inhibiting effect of oxygen was observed in both alcohol-producing and lactate-producing fermentation and is now known as the "Pasteur effect." In later years, a similar effect was observed in skeletal muscle, where lactate production was enhanced by an anaerobic environment and diminished by an aerobic environment (2).

The observation that a lack of oxygen is associated with an increase in lactate production has been misinterpreted as meaning that increased lactate production is evidence of a lack of oxygen. However, lactate can be produced in large quantities under aerobic conditions. To understand the mechanisms for aerobioc lactate production, it is necessary to review the reactions involved in glucose metabolism.

Glucose Metabolism

The metabolism of glucose is outlined in Figure 4.1. There are two general pathways for glucose breakdown: one is located in the cytoplasm (and is known as *glycolysis*), and the other is located in mitochondria. The glycolytic pathway operates in the presence or absence of oxygen, and has an energy yield of 2 ATP molecules per glucose molecule, while the mitochondrial pathway proceeds only in the presence of oxygen, and has an energy yield of 30 ATP molecules per glucose molecule.

The breakdown of the glucose molecule begins in the cytoplasm, and reaches a pivotal point with the formation of two pyruvate molecules. (Pyruvate is the conjugate base of pyruvic acid, which readily dissociates.) When oxygenation is adequate, pyruvate moves into mitochondria and provides the optimal energy yield for glucose metabolism (32 ATP molecules per glucose molecule). Note in Figure 4.1 that oxygen is not directly involved in the oxidative breakdown of glucose metabolites in the mitochondria. This is accomplished by oxidation reactions in the Krebs cycle (remem-

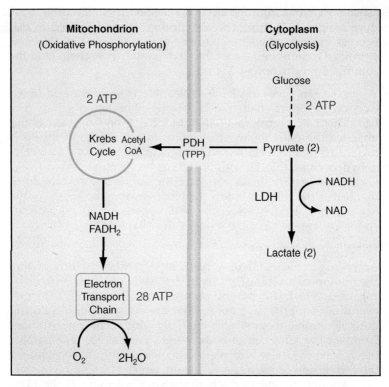

FIGURE 4.1 The pathways of glucose metabolism. ATP = adenosine tri-phosphate, PDH = pyruvate dehydrogenase, TPP = thiamine pyrophosphate, LDH = lactate dehydrogenase, NAD and NADH = nicotinamide adenine dinucleotide (oxidized and reduced), FADH$_2$ = flavin adenine dinucleotide (reduced). See text for further explanation.

ber that oxidation involves the loss of electrons, and reduction involves the addition of electrons); the released electrons are then added to the the coenzymes NAD and FAD. The reduced coenzymes (NADH and FADH$_2$) serve as electron carriers and travel to the inner mitochondrial membrane, where they donate their electrons to the first in a series of four protein complexes (i.e., the *electron transport chain*). The electrons are then passed from one protein complex to the next, and this transfer results in the production of energy-storing ATP molecules (a process is known as *oxidative phosphorylation.*) The final protein complex (cytochrome oxidase) is a heme-containing protein that binds oxygen, and the "spent" electrons from the electron transport chain are used to reduce oxygen to water. (The chemical reactions involved in this process are presented in Chapter 8.) This removal of electrons permits the continued use of the electron transport chain (and the continued production of ATP).

When oxygen is not available to clear electrons at the end of the electron transport chain, oxidative phosphorylation grinds to a halt. This has a retrograde effect that halts the Krebs cycle and impedes the entry of pyruvate into mitochondria. Pyruvate is then converted to lactate via a reaction that is catalyzed by lactate dehydrogenase (LDH), with NADH as the electron donor. (*Note:* Lactic acid readily dissociates, and the lactate anion is the form that leaves the cell and enters the bloodstream. The source of the extracellular acidosis associated with hyperlactatemia is a debated topic that is beyond the scope of this chapter.)

Aerobic Lactate Production

According to the metabolic scheme just described (which mirrors the traditional teaching), pyruvate is the end point of aerobic glycolysis, and lactate is the end point of anaerobic glycolysis. However, this is not the case, because lactate is also produced during normal, aerobic metabolism: the daily production rate is about 20 mmol per kilogram of body weight per day (3). The aerobic production of lactate is attributed to the equilibrium constant for the conversion of pyruvate to lactate, which strongly favors lactate production, and to the high enzymatic activity of the LDH isoform that facilitates the reaction. The favored production of lactate is evident in the extracellular lactate:pyruvate ratios, which are 23:1 in the brain, 10-13:1 in skeletal muscle, and 7:1 in the liver (4).

Aerobic Hyperlactatemia

The ability to produce lactate aerobically means that an increase in the blood lactate concentration (hyperlactatemia) is not necessarily a reflection of tissue hypoxia. In fact, there are numerous instances in which hyperlactatemia develops in the setting of adequate tissue oxygenation. The notable sources of "aerobic hyperlactatemia" are listed in Table 4.1. The source that deserves special attention is sepsis and septic shock (highlighted in red), because these conditions are the leading cause of in-hospital deaths in the United States (5) and the leading cause of death worldwide (6). The following is a brief review of the evidence that hyperlactatemia in sepsis and septic shock is aerobic in origin.

TABLE 4.1	Sources of Aerobic Hyperlactatemia
Conditions	**Drugs and Toxins**
Asthma (severe)	β Agonists
Ketoacidosis	Cyanide
Liver Dysfunction	Metformin
Seizures	Propofol
Sepsis/Septic Shock	Propylene Glycol
Thiamine Deficiency	Salicylates
Tumors	Toxic Alcohols

Sepsis and Septic Shock

The plasma lactate level plays an important role in the diagnosis, management, and prognosis of sepsis and septic shock. Sepsis is defined as a dysregulated host response to infection that results in life-threatening organ dysfunction, while septic shock is a subset of sepsis that is identified by volume-insensitive hypotension and hyperlactatemia (i.e., serum lactate > 2 mmol/L) (7). According to these definitions, hyperlactatemia is a universal consequence of septic shock. It is also a frequent finding in cases of sepsis without septic shock, and serum lactate measurements have been adopted as a screening tool for the early detection of sepsis (8). In addition to its diagnostic value, hyperlactatemia has prognostic significance in sepsis and septic shock. The risk of a fatal outcome in these conditions is directly related to the presence and severity of hyperlactatemia (9) and to the length of time required for lactate levels to return to normal after treatment is initiated (i.e., the longer the time to normalization, the greater the mortality risk) (10). This latter observation has led to the use of lactate-guided treatment protocols for sepsis and septic shock (11).

The correlation between lactate levels and mortality rates has been used as evidence that tissue hypoxia is the cause of death in sepsis and septic shock. However, the following observations do not support this contention.

Tissue Oxygenation

In an animal model of sepsis, the use of a positron-emitting marker of hypoxia (18F-fluoromisonidazole) showed no evidence of cellular hypoxia in any of the organs studied, which included the brain, heart, lungs, and skeletal muscle (12). In human studies, direct recordings of the PO_2 in skeletal muscle have shown that the tissue PO_2 is actually *increased* in sepsis and septic shock (13,14). The results of one of these studies is shown in Figure 4.2 (13). In this case, the PO_2 in the brachoradialis muscle (in the forearm) was recorded in three groups of subjects: healthy volunteers, patients in the immediate period following cardiopulmonary bypass surgery, and patients with septic shock. The skeletal muscle PO_2 was equivalent in the healthy subjects and the postoperative patients, but it was almost three fold higher in the patients with

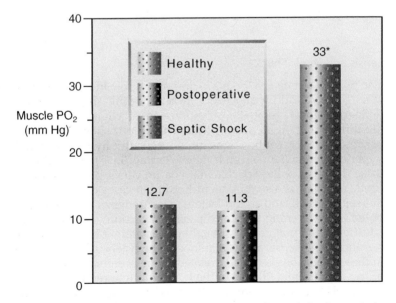

FIGURE 4.2 A comparison of PO_2 recordings from skeletal muscle in healthy volunteers, postoperative patients following major surgery, and patients with septic shock. The numbers above the bars indicate the mean PO_2 for each study group, and the asterisk indicates a significant difference (p<0.001) from the other groups. Data from Reference 13.

septic shock. (It is worth noting that most of the patients with septic shock in this study did not survive the illness.) A similar study in patients with sepsis showed a direct correlation between the magnitude of increase in skeletal muscle PO_2 and the severity of illness (14). The increase in tissue PO_2 in sepsis is consistent with the theory that mitochondrial utilization of O_2 is defective in sepsis; a condition known as *cytopathic hypoxia* (15).

Pyruvate Dehydrogenase

The pyruvate dehydrogenase (PDH) enzyme is involved in the oxidative conversion of pyruvate to acetyl coenzyme A (acetyl CoA); a reaction that requires thiamine pyrophosphate as a cofactor (see Figure 4.1). This reaction moves glycolysis into mitochondria, which allows for complete oxidation of the glucose substrate. Sepsis has been shown to depress PDH activity (16); an action attributed to bacterial toxins (e.g., endotoxin) and proinflammatory cytokines (e.g., TNFα) (2,17). This results in glycolysis being diverted to lactate production, which produces hyperlactatemia that is not the result of tissue hypoxia (16). Inhibition of PDH is one mechanism for the proposed defect in mitochondrial O_2 utilization in sepsis (i.e., cytopathic hypoxia).

Dichloroacetate (DCA) is an activator of PDH that is effective only when oxygenation is adequate. Both animal and human studies have shown that DCA reduces serum lactate levels in sepsis (18,19), and this provides further evidence that tissue hypoxia is not a feature of sepsis. The actions of DCA are demonstrated in Figure 4.3 (18). In this case, an endotoxin-induced increase in the serum lactate level was completely reversed by administration of DCA. Note also that inhalation of a 12% O_2 mixture (hypoxic challenge) did not increase the serum lactate level. These results clearly demonstrate the disconnect between increases in serum lactate and tissue hypoxia.

Thiamine Deficiency

Thiamine pyrophosphate is a cofactor for the PDH enzyme (see Figure 4.1), and thiamine deficiency is a recognized cause of hyperlactatemia in the absence of cellular hypoxia (20). Thiamine deficiency has been demonstrated in up to 20% of patients with septic shock (21), and intravenous thiamine administration has been shown to reduce serum lactate levels in this condition (22). Therefore, thiamine deficiency is a potential (and often overlooked) source of aerobic hyperlactatemia.

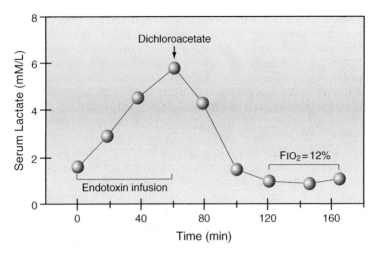

FIGURE 4.3 The effects of endotoxin, dichloroacetate, and inhalation of 12% O_2 (hypoxic challenge) on serum lactate levels. Data from Reference 18.

Nitric Oxide

The inflammatory response that accompanies sepsis is associated with increased production of nitric oxide, a reactive free radical that has multiple roles in sepsis (including the vasodilation that is characteristic of sepsis). Nitric oxide is a well-known source of mitochondrial dysfunction because of its ability to inhibit cytochrome oxidase (the last component of the electron transport chain), thereby interfering with oxidative phosphorylation (23). In addition, nitric oxide readily reacts with superoxide radicals (which are abundant in sites of inflammation) to produce peroxynitrite, a potent inhibitor of the electron transport system in mitochondria (23). (The reaction of nitric oxide with superoxide radicals is detailed in Chapter 8.) The combined effects of nitric oxide and peroxynitrite represent an important source of the mitochondrial dysfunction in sepsis.

Increased Glycolysis

Stressful conditions like sepsis are accompanied by an accumulation of the glucose transporter protein at the cell surface, which increases glucose uptake into cells (24). This results in a 40-50% increase in the rate of glycolysis during sepsis, and a similar increase in lactate and pyruvate release from cells (12). (The equivalent release of lactate and pyruvate is evidence of aerobic glycolysis.)

The enhanced glycolysis during sepsis is attributed to stimulation of β-2 adrenergic receptors by circulating catecholamines, especially epinephrine (25). This ability of sepsis to increase the rate of glycolysis, while also inhibiting pyruvate movement into mitochondria, is the principal engine for aerobic hyperlactatemia.

Summary

There is considerable evidence showing that the hyperlactatemia in sepsis and septic shock is a result in a defect in O_2 utilization by mitochondria, and not a defect in O_2 availability. The mitochondrial dysfunction in sepsis is attributed to several factors, including inhibition of the pyruvate dehydrogenase enzyme (e.g., by bacterial products and thiamine deficiency) and inhibition of the electron transport chain (e.g., by nitric oxide). This mitochondrial dysfunction, combined with a stress-induced increase in glycolysis, leads to an increase in lactate production that is aerobic in origin.

How Common is Anaerobic Lactate Production?

Anaerobic production of lactate occurs only when oxygen levels are insufficient to support ATP production in mitochondria. What seems relevant in this regard is the evidence presented in Chapter 3 (see the section on "Critical PO_2") that ATP production can continue until the PO_2 drops below 0.5 mm Hg. This suggests that anaerobic lactate production is likely to be an uncommon event; a notion supported by animal studies showing that cellular ATP levels remain unchanged in conditions believed to produce tissue hypoxia, such as ischemia and severe hypoxemia (26). Observations like these have led to a "paradigm shift" in the perceived role of anaerobiosis as a source of hyperlactatemia, as highlighted in the following statement:

> Today, it is well established that any increase in lactate concentration typically represents something other than O_2 limitation; hypoxia-driven lactate accumulation is very much the exception rather than the rule. (2)

Lactate as an Oxidative Fuel

The emerging consensus is that lactate is not a waste product of anaerobic metabolism, but instead serves as an alternative fuel source during periods of metabolic stress (2,25,27). A comparison of the energy yield from the oxidation of glucose and lactate is shown in Table 4.2. On a molecular basis, the energy yield from

Table 4.2   Lactate vs. Glucose as Oxidative Fuels

Substrate	Molecular Weight	Energy Yield	Caloric Density
Glucose	180 g/mol	673 kcal/mol	3.74 kcal/g
Lactate	90 g/mol	326 kcal/mol	3.62 kcal/g
Lactate x 2	180 g/mol	652 kcal/mol	

glucose is about twice that of lactate, but one glucose molecule produces two molecules of lactate, so the overall energy yield from lactate production is similar to that of glucose. The caloric density for glucose and lactate shown in Table 4.2 (3.74 vs. 3.62 kcal/g) indicates that *lactate is equivalent to glucose as an oxidative fuel.*

Lactate Shuttles

Lactate can serve as a source of energy when glucose availability is threatened by heightened metabolic demands. The transfer of lactate from a site of increased production is called a *lactate shuttle* (27). The first demonstrated lactate shuttle involved the transport of lactate from skeletal muscle to liver, where lactate is used as a substrate for gluconeogenesis. (The subsequent use of glucose to generate lactate completes what is known as the *Cori cycle.*) Lactate can also be shuttled for use as an oxidative fuel; this typically requires a conversion of lactate to pyruvate, which then enters the mitochondrion for oxidative phosphorylation. This type of shuttle can involve distant organs, or cells within the same organ. This latter phenomenon (an intraorgan lactate shuttle) has been demonstrated in exercising muscle, where the lactate produced in white "glycolytic" muscle fibers is shuttled to red "oxidative" muscle fibers (27). During exercise, about 75% of the lactate produced serves as an oxidative fuel, while 25% is used for gluconeogenesis (27).

In conditions of metabolic stress, lactate is often used as an oxidative fuel by the heart and brain. In this situation, lactate can provide 60% of the energy needs of the myocardium (2), and there is evidence that lactate improves cardiac performance in circulatory shock (28). Lactate can also provide about 25–30% of the energy needs of the brain in stressful conditions (29), and the brain is equipped with its own intraorgan lactate shuttle, where astro-cytes transfer their lactate to neurons for oxidative energy (2). Ad-aptations like these help to preserve the viability of the heart and brain in life-threatening conditions.

OXYGEN DEBT

Another popular marker of tissue hypoxia is an oxygen consump-tion (VO_2) that is below normal (in the absence of hypothermia); the cumulative deficit in VO_2 is known as the *oxygen debt* (30). The whole-body VO_2 can be measured as the difference in O_2 con-centration between inhaled and exhaled gas over a specified time period, or it can be calculated using a modified Fick equation; i.e.,

$$VO_2 = Q \times (CaO_2 - CvO_2) \qquad (4.1)$$

where Q is the volumetric flow rate (cardiac output), and ($CaO_2 - CvO_2$) is the difference in O_2 content between arterial and mixed venous (pulmonary artery) blood. This calculation typical-ly requires measurements obtained with a pulmonary artery bal-loon flotation catheter.

Origin

The concept of oxygen debt was introduced in the 1920s to explain the hypermetabolism that follows a period of strenuous exercise (31). According to this concept, the exercise-induced increase in serum lactate levels is a reflection of anaerobic metabolism (the oxygen debt), and post exercise increase in VO_2 is a mechanism for "repaying the oxygen debt." This concept generated a Nobel Prize for its originator (the British physiologist, A.V. Hill), and it remained unchallenged for almost 50 years, until a study in 1971 showed that the post exercise increase in VO_2 is the result of an increase in body temperature (32). Studies show that the O_2 levels in skeletal muscle remain unchanged as lactate produc-tion steadily rises during muscle contraction and graded exercise (33,34), indicating that there is no period of anaerobic metabolism during exercise (and hence no oxygen debt).

Clinical Applications

A clinical example of an oxygen debt is shown in Figure 4.4. In this case, a patient who underwent abdominal aortic aneurysm repair developed an early and persistent decrease in VO_2 that was below the lower limit of normal (the dotted line). The shaded area shows the magnitude and duration of the VO_2 deficit, and represents the oxygen debt. (Note that the decrease in VO_2 occurs before the appearance of hyperlactatemia, suggesting that the decrease in VO_2 is the source of the elevated serum lactate levels.) Clinical studies have shown that patients who develop a persistent O_2 debt following surgery are more likely to develop postoperative multiorgan failure (30). This same correlation has been observed in patients with circulatory shock.

The adoption of the oxygen debt concept in clinical medicine is based on the assumption that an abnormally low VO_2 is evidence of tissue hypoxia. However, it is also possible that a subnormal VO_2 can be the result of a decrease in O_2 utilization in mitochondria (mitochondrial dysfunction), without a decrease in O_2 availability. (In the case depicted in Figure 4.4, the postoperative decline in VO_2 could be the result of nitric oxide-induced inhibition of the electron transport chain, as a consequence of the inflammation that accompanies major surgery.) Thus, the O_2 debt is not necessarily a marker of tissue hypoxia. It is, however, a marker of a cellular energy deficit, which is why the O_2 debt has the prognostic value mentioned earlier.

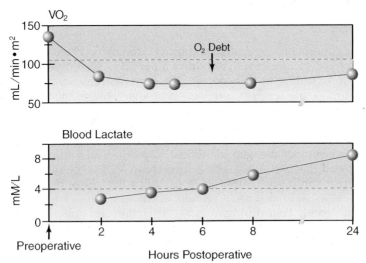

FIGURE 4.4 Serial measurements of whole-body O_2 consumption (VO_2) and serum lactate levels in the postoperative period following an abdominal aortic aneurysm repair. The dotted lines indicate the upper (for lactate) and lower (for VO_2) limits of normal. The shaded area represents the oxygen debt. Data from personal experience.

Focused Management

Clinical studies showing a correlation between the presence of an oxygen debt and the likelihood of multiorgan dysfunction led to management strategies that attempted to achieve normal or supranormal levels of VO_2 by promoting O_2 delivery to tissues. However, the impact of this approach on mortality rates was inconsistent, with individual studies showing either reduced mortality (35), no change in mortality (36), or increased mortality (37). As a result, the oxygen debt concept has largely been abandoned as a management strategy. Of interest, one of the cited shortcomings of this management strategy was the limited ability to increase the VO_2 to the desired level despite the imposed increase in O_2 delivery (36). This limited ability to influence the VO_2 is the central theme of the next two chapters.

SUMMATION

The perception that tissue hypoxia is a common cause of death is based primarily on studies that use hyperlactatemia and an oxygen debt as markers of tissue hypoxia. However, neither of these markers is specific for tissue hypoxia. In the case of hyperlactatemia, the emerging consensus is that lactate is not a waste product of anaerobic metabolism, but rather is an oxidative fuel that can be utilized during periods of metabolic stress.

Based on the information presented in this chapter, it is reasonable to conclude that tissue hypoxia is NOT a common prelude to death. In fact, considering the damaging effects of oxygen and its reactive derivatives (presented in the second section of the book), it may be that the *presence* of oxygen is the real threat to life.

REFERENCES

a. Newland, S., How We Die: Reflections on Life's Final Chapter. New York: Random House, 1994.

1. Barnett JA, Entian K-D. A history of research on yeasts, 9: regulation of sugar metabolism. Yeast 2005; 22:835-894.
2. Ferguson BS, Rogatzki MJ, Goodwin ML, et al. Lactate metabolism: historical context, prior misinterpretations, and current understanding. Europ J Appl Physiol 2018; 118:691-728.
3. Kraut JA, Madias NE. Lactic acidosis. N Engl J Med 2014; 371:2309-2319.
4. Rogatski MJ, Ferguson BS, Goodwin ML, Gladden LB. Lactate is al-

ways the end product of glycolysis. Front Neuroscience 2015; 9:1-7.

5. Liu V, Escobar GJ, Greene JD, et al. Hospital deaths in patients with sepsis from 2 independent cohorts. JAMA 2014; 312:90-92.

6. Rudd KE, Johnson SC, Agesa KM, et al. Global, regional, and national sepsis incidence and mortality, 1990-2017: analysis for the Global Burden of Disease Study. Lancet 2020; 395:200-211.

7. Singer M, Deutschman C, Seymore CW, et al. The third international consensus definitions of sepsis and septic shock. JAMA 2016; 315:801-810.

8. Contenti J, Corraze H, Lemoël F, Levraut J. Effectiveness of arterial, venous, and capillary blood lactate as a sepsis triage tool in ED patients. Am J Emerg Med 2015; 33:167-172.

9. Trzeciak S, Dellinger RP, Chansky ME, et al. Serum lactate as a predictor of mortality in patients with infection. Intensive Care Med 2007; 33:970–977.

10. Nguyen HB, Rivers EP, Knoblich BP, et al. Early lactate clearance is associated with improved outcome in severe sepsis and septic shock. Crit Care Med 2004; 32:1637–1642.

11. Jansen TC, van Bommel J, Schoonderbeek FJ, et al. Early lactate-guided therapy in intensive care unit patients: a multicenter, open-label, randomized controlled trial. Am J Resp Crit Care Med 2010; 182:753-761.

12. Hotchkiss RS, Karl IE. Reevaluation of the role of cellular hypoxia and bioenergetic failure in sepsis. JAMA 1992; 267:1503-1510.

13. Sair M, Etherington PJ, Winlove P, Evans TW. Tissue oxygenation and perfusion in patients with systemic sepsis. Crit Care Med 2001; 29:1343-1349.

14. Boekstegers P, Weidenhofer S, Kapsner T, Werdan K. Skeletal muscle partial pressure of oxygen in patients with sepsis. Crit Care Med 1994; 22:640-650.

15. Fink MP. Cytopathic hypoxia. Mitochondrial dysfunction as mechanism contributing to organ dysfunction in sepsis. Crit Care Clin 2001; 17:219–237.

16. Vary TC. Sepsis-induced alteration in pyruvate dehydrogenase complex activity in rat skeletal muscle: effects on plasma lactate. Shock 1996; 6:89-94.

17. Thomas GW, Mains CW, Slone DS, et al. Potential dysregulation of the pyruvate dehydrogenase complex by bacterial toxins and insulin. J Trauma 2009; 67:628-633.

18. Curtis SE, Cain SM. Regional and systemic oxygen delivery/uptake relations and lactate flux in hyperdynamic, endotoxin-treated dogs. Am Rev Respir Dis 1992; 145:348-354.

19. Stacpoole PW, Nagaraja NM, Hutson AD. Efficacy of dichloroacetate as a lactate-lowering drug. J Clin Pharmacol 2003; 43:683-691.

20. Oriot D, Wood C, Gottesman R, et al. Severe lactic acidosis related to acute thiamine deficiency. JPEN: J Parenter Enteral Nutr 1991; 15:105-109.

21. Donnino MW, Carney E, Cocchi MN, et al. Thiamine deficiency in critically ill patients with sepsis. J Crit Care 2010; 25:576-581.

22. Woolum JA, Abner EL, Kelly A, et al. Effect of thiamine administration on lactate clearance and mortality in patients with septic shock. Crit Care Med 2018; 46:1747-1752.

23. Cassina A, Radi R. Differential inhibitory action of nitric oxide and peroxynitrite on mitochondrial electron transport. Arch Biochem Biophy 1996; 328:309-316.

24. Windall CC, Baldwin SA, Davies A, et al. Cellular stress induces a redistribution of the glucose transporter protein. FASEB J 1990; 4:1634-1637.

25. Levy B. Lactate and the shock state: the metabolic view. Curr Opin Crit Care 2006; 12:315-321.

26. Gutierrez G, Pohil RJ, Andry JM, et al. Bioenergetics of rabbit skeletal muscle during hypoxemia and ischemia. J Appl Physiol 1988; 65:608-616.

27. Brooks GA. Cell-cell and intracellular lactate shuttles. J Physiol 2009; 587:5591-5600.

28. Kline JA, Thornton LR, Lopaschuk GD, et al. Lactate improves cardiac efficiency after hemorrhagic shock. Shock 2000; 14:215-221.

29. van Hall G, Strømstead M, Rasmussen P, et al. Blood lactate is an important energy source for the human brain. J Cereb Blood Flow Metab 2009; 29:1121-1129.

30. Shoemaker WC, Appel PL, Kram HB. Role of oxygen debt in the development of organ failure, sepsis, and death in high-risk surgical patients. Chest 1992; 102:208-215.

31. Hill AV, Long CNH, Lupton H. Muscular exercise, lactic acid, and supply and utilization of oxygen. IV. The oxygen debt at the end of exercise. Proc R Soc Lond B Biol Sci 1924; 97:127-137.

32. Brooks GA, Hittelman KJ, Faulkner JA, Beyer RE. Temperature, skeletal muscle mitochondrial function, and oxygen debt. Am J Physiol 1971; 220:1053-1059.

33. Connett RJ, Gayeski TE, Honig CR. Lactate efflux is unrelated to intracellular PO_2 in a working red muscle in situ. J Appl Physiol 1986; 61:402-408.

34. Richardson RS, Norszewski EA, Leigh JS, Wagner PD. Lactate efflux from exercising human skeletal muscle: role of intracellular PO_2. J Appl Physiol 1998; 85:627-634.

35. Shoemaker WC, Appel P, Kram H, et al. Prospective trial of supranormal values of survivors as therapeutic goals in high-risk surgical patients. Chest 1988; 94:1176-1186.

36. Yu M, Levy M, Smith P, et al. Effect of maximizing oxygen delivery on morbidity and mortality in critically ill patients. A prospective, randomized, controlled trial. Crit Care Med 1993; 21:830-838.

37. Hayes M, Timmin A, Yau EHS, et al. Elevation of systemic oxygen delivery in the treatment of critically ill patients. N Engl J Med 1994; 330:1717-1722.

Is oxygen therapy based on tissue needs?

5

"It is what we think we know already that often prevents us from learning."

Claude Bernard (1813-1878)

There is a fondness for oxygen therapy that is unmatched by any other treatment modality, and this sentiment is expressed by the liberal and unregulated use of oxygen in modern clinical practice. The popularity of oxygen therapy is readily apparent in emergency rooms (where inhaled O_2 is a knee-jerk response to acute illness) and in intensive care units (where a patient who is not connected to a source of oxygen is a rare sight). Inhaled oxygen is also available to the general public in "oxygen bars" (where pure oxygen is delivered through nasal prongs, in a variety of scents) and in portable canisters that deliver oxygen sprays (for a quick "pick-me-up").

This unbridled use of oxygen deserves scrutiny, especially in light of the information in Chapter 3 showing that parenchymal cells normally operate in an oxygen-poor environment, and that oxidative metabolism can continue at PO_2 levels down to 1 mm Hg and even lower. This chapter provides some of this scrutiny, with a focus on the relationship between oxygen use and oxygen need.

CURRENT GUIDELINES

Despite the widespread use of oxygen therapy, there are surprisingly few guidelines for this practice. The first expert-driven guideline for O_2 therapy was published in 1984 (1), and the principal recommendation was stated as follows:

> "Supplemental oxygen therapy is appropriate in acute conditions when there is laboratory documentation of an arterial PO_2 (PaO_2) <60 mm Hg or an arterial O_2 saturation (SaO_2) <90 %; *tissue hypoxia is commonly assumed to be present at these laboratory values*" (italics mine)."

This statement is consistent with the consensus definition of hypoxemia as a PaO_2 <60 mm Hg or an SaO_2 <90%, and this threshold for O_2 therapy has changed little over the years. More recent guidelines include a ceiling for O_2 therapy, in recognition of the

55

toxic potential of oxygen. The most recent recommendations for O_2 therapy (2) include a target SaO_2 of 88-92% for patients at risk of CO_2 retention and an SaO_2 of 90-94% for most other patients.

The major issue with the recommendations for O_2 therapy is the assumption that tissue oxygenation is threatened or compromised when the PaO_2 falls below 60 mm Hg, or the SaO_2 falls below 90%. This is addressed later in the chapter. An additional concern is the preferred use of the SaO_2 as a guide for O_2 therapy (see next).

The SaO_2

The introduction of pulse oximetry in the 1970s provided a reliable, noninvasive method of monitoring the SaO_2 at the bedside. Over the ensuing decade, the use of pulse oximetry became so widespread that the SaO_2 was referred to as "the fifth vital sign" (3). Because of the availability and ease of recording, the SaO_2 has become the preferred measure for guiding O_2 therapy. However, the driving force for the movement of O_2 into tissues is the PO_2 gradient from blood to tissues, so the PaO_2 is a more appropriate measure for guiding O_2 therapy.

Oxyhemoglobin Dissociation Curve

The SaO_2 can be misleading when pulse oximetry recordings are suboptimal (which occurs more often than suspected) (4), and when there are shifts in the oxyhemoglobin dissociation curve. The latter influence is shown in Figure 5.1. The oxyhemoglobin dissociation curve describes the relationship between the PaO_2 and the SaO_2; a leftward shift in the curve increases the SaO_2 at any given PaO_2 (which means Hb is less likely to release O_2 into the tissues), while a rightward shift has the opposite effect. To appreciate the misleading influence of these shifts, consider that an increase in SaO_2 usually indicates that more O_2 is available for the tissues, but if the increase is due to a leftward shift in the oxyhemoglobin dissociation curve, then less O_2 is available for the tissues. The conditions that produce shifts in the oxyhemoglobin dissociation curve are shown in Figure 5.1.

Noncompliance

There is a general lack of regard for published guidelines on O_2 therapy. In a review of 11 studies that evaluated compliance with published guidelines (5), compliance rates varied from zero to 55%, and five studies showed a compliance rate below 10% . Each

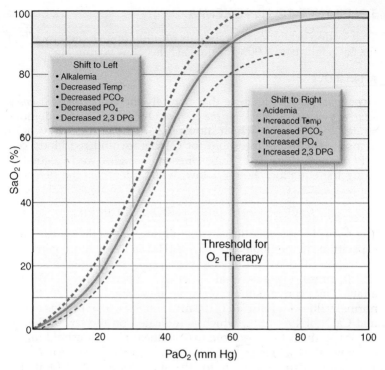

FIGURE 5.1 Oxyhemoglobin dissociation curves. When the normal curve (solid line) is shifted to the left or right (dotted lines), the relationship between the PaO_2 and SaO_2 is altered. See text for further explanation.

of these studies included an educational initiative to improve acceptance of the guidelines, but compliance rates typically remained below 50% despite the educational effort. Noncompliance with guidelines is certainly a factor in the reported overuse of O_2 therapy (6).

The misuse of oxygen mostly involves a disregard for the recommended ceiling level of SaO_2 or PaO_2; e.g., in a multicenter study that evaluated 107,000 arterial blood gas results in patients receiving O_2 therapy, three-quarters of the samples showed a PaO_2 or SaO_2 that exceeded the recommended target range (7). This indicates a disturbing lack of concern for the damaging effects of oxygen, and implies that the current use of O_2 therapy is not only excessive, it's also dangerous.

TOLERANCE TO HYPOXEMIA

This section examines the rationale for initiating O_2 therapy when the SaO_2 falls below 90%, or the PaO_2 is below 60 mm Hg.

Arterial O_2 Content

Hypoxemia has one feature that is rarely mentioned; i.e., it *has a relatively minor influence on the arterial O_2 content*. This is demonstrated in Figure 5.2, which shows the arterial O_2 content (CaO_2) associated with the threshold for O_2 therapy and red blood cell (RBC) transfusions. The CaO_2 values in this figure were calculated using the equation shown below, which identifies the determinants of CaO_2.

$$CaO_2 = 1.34 \times [Hb] \times SaO_2 \times 10 \ (mL/L) \qquad (5.1)$$

The terms in this equation are as follows: 1.34 is the O_2 carrying capacity of hemoglobin (in mL/g), [Hb] is the hemoglobin concentration (in g/100 mL), SaO_2 is arterial oxyhemoglobin saturation (expressed as a decimal rather than a percentage), and 10 is a factor that converts the CaO_2 from mL/100 mL to mL/L. Using normal values for [Hb] (15 g/100 mL) and SaO_2 (0.98) yields a normal CaO_2 of 197 mL/L, which is indicated on the left in Figure 5.2. When the SaO_2 is reduced to 0.90 (the typical threshold for O_2 therapy), the CaO_2 is 181 mL/L, which is an 8% decrease in CaO_2. Therefore, a drop in SaO_2 to the threshold for initiating O_2 therapy results in a relatively small (8%) decrease in the O_2 content of blood, and this minor change seems unlikely to influence tissue oxygenation.

For RBC transfusions, the recommended transfusion trigger is a Hb level of 7 g/dL (see Chapter 6), and this value yields a CaO_2 of 92 mL/L, which is a 64% decrease from baseline. Therefore, there is a large discrepancy between the arterial O_2 content that triggers O_2 therapy (181 mL/L) and the one that triggers RBC transfusions. (92 mL/L). Since tissue oxygenation is not compromised at an arterial O_2 content of 92 mL/L, this is evidence that oxygen therapy is initiated when tissue oxygenation is adequate.

Hypobaric Hypoxemia

Human studies of severe hypoxemia have been conducted mostly in decompression chambers, where subjects are exposed to low atmospheric pressures. This condition is known as *hypobaric hypoxia*, and the resulting decrease in arterial oxygenation is called *hypobaric hypoxemia*. The ability to tolerate severe hypobaric hy-

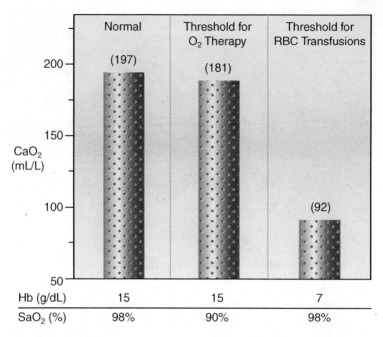

FIGURE 5.2 Bar graph showing the relationship between the arterial O_2 content (CaO_2) and the thresholds for O_2 therapy ($SaO_2 = 90\%$) and RBC transfusions (Hb = 7 g/dL). The numbers in parentheses are calculated CaO_2 values based on the corresponding hemoglobin (Hb) and arterial oxyhemoglobin saturation (SaO_2) values shown below the graph.

poxemia was first demonstrated "in the field" by an intrepid Italian mountaineer named Reinhold Messner.

Reinhold Messner

Reinhold Messner is the most accomplished mountaineer in the history of the discipline. One of his most notable accomplishments occurred in 1978, when he and fellow climber Peter Habeler reached the summit of Mount Everest (elevation 29,029 feet,) without the use of supplemental oxygen (see Fig. 5.3). Messner is a naturalist who believes that scaling mountains should be experienced with as few artificial aids as possible, and he eschewed the use of "artificial oxygen aids" throughout his career. Prior to his historic climb, Messner was warned (by experts of the time) that reaching the summit of Mount Everest without inhaled O_2 was suicidal; he would lose consciousness and suffer permanent brain

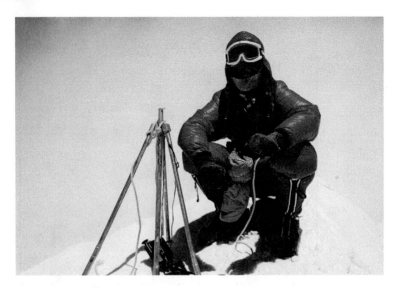

FIGURE 5.3 Reinhold Messner at the summit of Mount Everest without an oxygen mask. The inhaled PO_2 at this altitude is only 43 mm Hg.

damage above an altitude of 26,000 feet (a region known as the "death zone"). However, this was an untested claim (like many others about oxygen), so Messner devised a simple test. Using a plane with a depressurized cabin, he was flown to an altitude just above the summit of Mount Everest while breathing ambient air. To the chagrin of many, Messner felt no ill effects as the plane climbed above 26,000 feet (the death zone) and reached a peak altitude of 30,000 feet. He later wrote, "I had seen the flight through without an oxygen mask, and I was still able to talk, to think, to sense everything" (8).

Thus did Reinhold Messner debunk one of the popular credos about the inability to survive in a low-O_2 environment. He went on to become the first to successfully climb all 14 mountains that exceed 8,000 meters (26,250 ft) in height, and he did it all without using supplemental O_2. (*Note:* There have been 198 successful ascents of Mount Everest without the use of oxygen. A list of the individuals who completed this task is available at www.8000ers.com.)

There were no physiological measurements obtained on Reinhold Messner at the summit of Mount Everest, but the degree of hypobaric hypoxia he faced can be determined by calculating the inhaled PO_2 (P_{IO_2}) at that elevation:

$$P_{IO_2} = (P_B - P_{H_2O}) \times 0.21 \qquad (5.2)$$

where P_B is the barometric pressure, P_{H_2O} is the pressure of water vapor (which accounts for the humidification of inhaled gases), and 0.21 is the fractional concentration of O_2 in the atmosphere. The P_B at the summit of Mount Everest is 253 mm Hg (9), or about one-third of the P_B at sea level (760 mm Hg), and the P_{H_2O} is 47 mm Hg, so the P_{IO_2} is $(253 - 47) \times 0.21 = 43$ mm Hg. This means that the inhaled PO_2 at the top of Mount Everest is lower than the arterial PO_2 that triggers O_2 therapy!

Severe Hypoxemia

The most influential of the decompression chamber studies is Operation Everest II (10), a simulated climb of Mount Everest that involved eight healthy volunteers (nonclimbers) who spent 40 days in a decompression chamber. During this time, the pressure in the chamber was gradually decreased until the P_{IO_2} reached 43 mm Hg, to replicate the P_{IO_2} at the summit of Mount Everest. The data from this study are shown in Table 5.1. Note the severity of the hypoxemia ($PaO_2 = 30$ mm Hg, $SaO_2 = 58\%$), but more importantly, note that there was no associated decrease in whole-body O_2 consumption and no increase in the plasma lactate level. These data demonstrate that aerobic metabolism is maintained at levels of hypoxemia that are rarely encountered (or allowed to persist) in clinical practice. (*Note:* The reliability of the lactate level as a marker of anaerobic metabolism is discussed in Chapter 4.)

More severe levels of hypobaric hypoxemia have been reported in the only study involving climbers on Mount Everest (11). Blood samples from four subjects breathing ambient air at an altitude of 27,559 ft (1,470 ft below the summit) showed a PaO_2 of 24.6 mm Hg, an SaO_2 of 54%, and a serum lactate of 2.2 mmol/L (mean values). Similar to the studies in decompression chambers, there was no evidence of impaired tissue oxygenation.

Acclimatization

Tolerance to severe hypobaric hypoxemia must be interpreted in light of the acclimatization response, which involves an increase in hemoglobin concentration that gradually develops over 3–4 weeks of exposure to low atmospheric pressures. This improves exercise performance (similar to "blood doping," but intrinsic in nature), which is attributed to improved O_2 delivery to tissues.

Table 5.1	Severe Hypobaric Hypoxemia		
	Sea Level	Summit of Mt. Everest	% Change
P_{IO_2} (mm Hg)	150	43	-73%
PaO_2 (mm Hg)	99	30	-70%
SaO_2 (%)	98	58	-41%
CaO_2 (mL/L)	179	119	-34%
VO_2 (mL/min)	350	386	+10%
VCO_2 (mL/min)	278	369	+33%
Lactate (mmol/L)	1.1	1.7	+55%

Numbers represent mean values, rounded to the nearest whole number (except lactate). P_{IO_2} = inhaled PO_2, CaO_2 = arterial O_2 content, VO_2 = O_2 consumption, VCO_2 = CO_2 production. Data from Reference 10.

However, there may be another process involved in the benefits of acclimatization, as explained next.

CO₂ Removal

The data in Table 5.1 show a 33% increase in CO_2 production (VCO_2) and a much smaller (10%) increase in O_2 consumption (VO_2) in these acclimatized subjects. The increase in VCO_2 is thus three times greater than the increase in VO_2, so the increase in CO_2 transport should be three times greater than the increase in O_2 transport. Since hemoglobin plays a major role in CO_2 transport (see Chapter 2), it is possible that the increase in hemoglobin concentration during acclimatization is more of a response to the greater needs of CO_2 transport. Carbon dioxide is an acid, so the enhanced CO_2 transport will help to alleviate acid buildup in the tissues, and this could contribute to the benefits of acclimatization.

Normobaric Hypoxemia

The hypoxemia encountered in clinical practice (*normobaric hypoxemia*) is almost always the result of a gas exchange abnormality in the lungs. There is limited information on tolerance to to this type of hypoxemia, primarily because it is corrected immediately, and not allowed to persist. The available information comes from small observational studies and case reports. The data in Table 5.2 are from a study of eight patients with acute respiratory failure who had a PaO_2 below 40 mm Hg while breathing room air for at least one hour (12). Shown in the table are the PaO_2, SaO_2, and plasma lactate level in each patient. There was no evidence of compromised tissue oxygenation in any patient, as determined by the normal lactate levels (≤2 mmol/L). Similar findings have been reported in individual case reports (13).

Organ Dysfunction

Organ dysfunction is used as (indirect) evidence of impaired aerobic metabolism from hypoxemia, and the organ most likely to be affected is the brain. Altered mentation is the most cited consequence of hypoxemia, but the severity of hypoxemia needed to alter brain function is not clear. There is a longstanding claim that organ dysfunction will not occur until the PaO_2 drops below

Table 5.2	Severe Normobaric Hypoxemia		
Patient	PaO_2 (mm Hg)	SaO_2 (%)	Lactate (mmol/L)
1	22	35	0.9
2	30	54	0.3
3	32	59	0.9
4	35	55	1.6
5	34	65	1.6
6	35	67	2.0
7	37	75	2.0
8	39	76	1.1

From Reference 12.

30 mm Hg, or the SaO_2 falls below 50% (14), but there is no evidence to support this claim. One observation that deserves mention is from a study where hypoxemia was not associated with mental status changes unless it was accompanied by heart failure (i.e., a low-flow state) (12). This suggests that hypoperfusion may be a greater threat to tissue oxygenation than hypoxemia. In fact, this would explain why there are conditions like hypovolemic shock and cardiogenic shock (i.e., low-flow shock), while "hypoxemic shock" is not a recognized clinical entity.

Summary

There are relatively few studies of tolerance to severe hypoxemia in humans, but the available evidence shows that aerobic metabolism is maintained at levels of SaO_2 and PaO_2 that are far below the threshold levels for O_2 therapy. This means that *O_2 therapy is commonly used when aerobic metabolism is NOT impaired*, and thus, *O_2 therapy is not based on tissue O_2 needs*.

RESPONSE TO O_2 THERAPY

This final section describes a peculiar feature of the physiological response to oxygen that has important implications.

Oxygen as Vasoconstrictor

Oxygen acts as a vasoconstrictor in all major organs except the lungs, where it acts as a vasodilator. This vasoconstrictor effect is demonstrated in Figure 5.4, which shows the density of open capillaries in an *in situ* skeletal muscle preparation as the surrounding PO_2 is increased from 5 to 150 mm Hg (15). Note that the capillary density steadily declines as the PO_2 rises, with no open capillaries visible at a PO_2 of 150 mm Hg. This progressive obliteration of capillaries has been observed in other studies (16) and is the result of vasoconstriction in small arterioles. The principal mechanism is loss of the vasodilating actions of nitric oxide (17), which is attributed to oxidation of nitric oxide by the superoxide radical, a "reactive oxygen species." (See Chapter 8 for more on this reaction.) There is evidence that vitamin C (a water-soluble antioxidant) eliminates the vasoconstrictor response to oxygen (18,19).

Coronary Circulation

Oxygen-induced vasoconstriction can produce significant decreases in coronary blood flow in patients with coronary artery disease (20). In the presence of stenotic lesions in the coronary arteries, this vasoconstrictor response can result in poststenotic

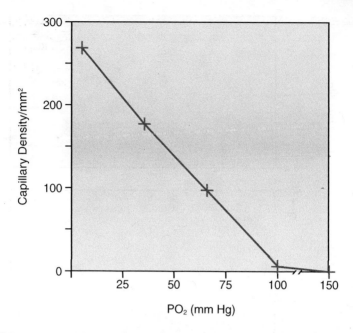

FIGURE 5.4 Capillary density in an *in situ* skeletal muscle preparation as the surrounding PO_2 is increased from 5 to 150 mm Hg. Data points represent mean values. Data from Reference 15.

myocardial deoxygenation (21), indicating that *O_2 therapy is a potential source of harm in acute coronary syndromes* (ACS). In recognition of this risk, the routine use of inhaled O_2 in ACS has been questioned. Several studies have shown no benefit from O_2 therapy in patients with ACS who are not hypoxemic (22). Based on these studies, the most recent guidelines on ST-elevation myocardial infarction (STEMI) includes a recommendation to restrict O_2 therapy to patients with hypoxemia (23). This recommendation, however, should include all patients with coronary artery disease.

Oxygen Transport

Oxygen-induced systemic vasoconstriction will increase left ventricular afterload, and this can result in a decrease in cardiac output (24). When this occurs, the ability of inhaled O_2 to augment systemic O_2 delivery will be curtailed. This is explained by the following equation for O_2 delivery (DO_2):

$$DO_2 = CO \times CaO_2 \qquad (5.3)$$

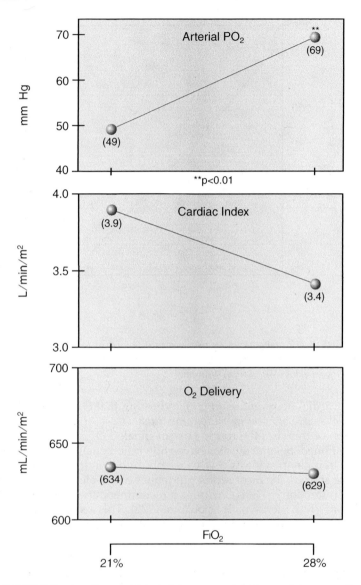

FIGURE 5.5 The effects of inhaled O_2 on arterial PO_2, cardiac output (indexed to body size), and systemic O_2 delivery in patients with acute exacerbation of COPD. Note that the the increase in arterial PO_2 is not accompanied by an increase in O_2 delivery because of the concurrent decrease in cardiac output. Data from Reference 24.

where CO is cardiac output, and CaO_2 is the arterial O_2 content (see Equation 5.1). This equation predicts that an increase in CaO_2 (from inhaled O_2) will increase systemic O_2 delivery, but a concurrent decrease in cardiac output will mitigate or eliminate this effect. This is demonstrated in Figure 5.5, which shows the response to inhaled O_2 in 20 patients with an acute exacerbation of COPD (24). Note that the increase in PaO_2 is accompanied by a proportional decrease in cardiac output, and the systemic O_2 delivery remains unchanged. This type of response would explain why inhaled O_2 has little or no influence on the whole-body O_2 consumption (25). It also demonstrates why *monitoring the PaO_2 or SaO_2 alone is inadequate for judging the response to inhaled O_2.*

Implications

There is a low-O_2 environment in tissues (see Chapter 3), which (from a teleological viewpoint) is a design advantage that limits the risk of oxidative tissue injury. The vasoconstrictor response to O_2 therapy serves as a protective mechanism that helps to maintain this advantage. The existence of such a response is thus a testament to the importance of maintaining a low-O_2 environment in tissues (and the protection from oxidative damage). Stated in more colloquial terms:

> "The tissues don't have much oxygen,
> and they want to keep it that way."

Adherence to this concept will discourage efforts to increase systemic O_2 delivery when tissue oxygenation is adequate, which is a common occurence with the current practice of O_2 therapy.

SUMMATION

The traditional threshold for O_2 therapy (SaO_2 <90%) was first proposed about 37 years ago and was not selected because of experimental data, but rather because of an assumption that tissue hypoxia will develop when the SaO_2 is lower than the threshold level. Since that time, studies of severe hypoxemia have shown that aerobic metabolism is maintained at SaO_2 levels that are far below the threshold for O_2 therapy. This means that O_2 therapy is initiated when it is not needed; i.e., *O_2 therapy is not based on tissue O_2 needs.*

The vasoconstrictor response to O_2 can be viewed as a mechanism for protecting tissues from exposure to excess O_2. The existence of such a response supports the notion (proposed in Chapter 3) that the low-O_2 environment in tissues is a design advantage that limits the risk of oxidative tissue injury.

REFERENCES

1. Fulmer JD, Snider GL. ACCP-NHLBI National Conference on Oxygen Therapy. Chest 1984; 86:234-247.

2. Siemieniuk RAC, Chu DK, Kim LH-Y, et al. Oxygen therapy for acutely ill medical patients: a clinical practice guideline. BMJ 2018; 363:k4169.

3. Mower WR, Myers G, Nicklin EL, et. al. Pulse oximetry as a fifth vital sign in emergency geriatric assessment. Acad Emerg Med 1998; 5:858–869.

4. Jubran A, Tobin M. Reliability of pulse oximetry in titrating supplemental oxygen therapy in ventilator-dependent patients. Chest 1990; 97:1420–1435.

5. Cousins JL, Wark PAB, McDonald VM. Acute oxygen therapy: a review of prescribing and delivery practice. Int J COPD 2016; 11:1067-1075.

6. Helmerhorst HJF, Schultz MJ, van der Voort PHJ, et al. Self-reported attitudes versus actual practice of oxygen therapy by ICU physicians and nurses. Ann Intensive Care 2014; 4:23.

7. Morgan DJ, Dhruva SS, Coon ER, et al. 2017 update on medical overuse: a systematic review. JAMA Intern Med 2018; 178:110-115.

8. Messner R. Last taboo: Everest without oxygen. In: Free Spirit: A Climber's Life. Seattle, WA: The Mountaineers, 1998:205-212.

9. West JB, Lahiri S, Maret KH, et al. Barometric pressures at extreme altitude on Mount Everest: physiological significance. J Appl Physiol 1983; 54:1188-1194.

10. Sutton JR, Reeves JT, Wagner PD, et al. Operation Everest II: oxygen transport during exercise at extreme simulated altitude. J Appl Physiol 1988; 1309-1321.

11. Grocott MP, Nartin DS, Levett DZ, et al. Arterial blood gases and oxygen content in climbers on Mount Everest. N Engl J Med 2009; 360:140-149.

12. Eldrigge FE. Blood lactate and pyruvate in pulmonary insufficiency. N Engl J Med 1966; 274:878-883.

13. Lundt T, Koller M, Kofstad J. Severe hypoxemia without evidence of tissue hypoxia in the adult respiratory distress syndrome. Crit Care Med 1984; 12:75-76.

14. Campbell EJM. Oxygen therapy in diseases of the chest. Br J Dis Chest 1964; 58:149-157.

15. Lindbolm L, Tuma RF, Arfors K-E. Influence of oxygen on perfused capillary density and red cell velocity in rabbit skeletal muscle. Microvasc Res 1980; 19:197-208.

16. Tsai AG, Cabrales P, Winslow RM, Intaglietta M. Microvascular oxygen distribution in awake hamster window chamber model during hyperoxia. Am J Physiol Heart Circ Physiol 2003; 285:H1537-1545.

17. Landmesser U, Harrison D, Drexler H. Oxidant stress – a major cause of reduced endothelial nitric oxide availability in cardiovascular disease. Eur J Clin Pharmacol 2006; 62:13-19.
18. Mak S, Egri Z, Tanna G, et al. Vitamin C prevents hyperoxia-mediated vasoconstriction and impairment of endothelium-dependent vasodilation. Am J Physiol Heart Circ Physiol 2002; 282:H2414-2421.
19. Gao Z, Spik S, Momen A, et al. Vitamin C prevents hyperoxia-mediated coronary vasoconstriction and impairment of myocardial function in healthy subjects. Eur J Appl Physiol 2012; 112:483-492.
20. Farquhar H, Weatherall M, Wijesinghe M, et al. Systematic review of studies of the effects of hyperoxia on coronary blood flow. Am Heart J 2009; 158:371-377.
21. Guensch DP, Fischer K, Yamaji K, et al. Effect of hyperoxia on myocardial oxygenation and function in patients with stable multivessel coronary artery disease. J Am Heart Assoc 2020; 9:e014739.
22. Khoshnood A. High time to omit oxygen therapy in ST elevation myocardial infarction. BMC Emerg Med 2018; 18:35.
23. Ibanez B, James S, Agewall S, et al. 2017 ESC Guidelines for the Management of Acute Myocardial Infarction in Patients Presenting With ST-segment Elevation: The Task Force for the Management of Acute Myocardial Infarction in Patients Presenting With ST-segment Elevation of the European Society of Cardiology (ESC) Eur Heart J 2018; 39:119-177.
24. DeGaute JP, Domengighetti G, Naeije R, et al. Oxygen delivery in acute exacerbation of chronic obstructive pulmonary disease. Effects of controlled oxygen therapy. Am Rev Respir Dis 1981; 124:26-30.
25. Lejeune P, Mols P, Naeije R, et al. Acute hemodynamic effects of controlled oxygen therapy in decompensated chronic obstructive pulmonary disease. Crit Care Med 1984; 12:1032–1035.

Are red blood cell transfusions based on tissue needs?

6

"A conscientious man would be cautious how he dealt in blood."

Edmund Burke (1729-1797)

The American Red Cross motto, *Blood Saves Lives*, is seared into the American psyche (its validity unquestioned), and this certainly plays a role in the estimated 36,000 red blood cell (RBC) transfusions given each day in the United States (1). The desired goal of RBC transfusions is to promote tissue oxygenation, but the actual goal is to increase the hemoglobin concentration and hematocrit (an effect that can also be achieved by changing body position, as shown in Fig. 6.1). This chapter examines the current practice of transfusing RBCs in the same manner that oxygen therapy was examined in the last chapter; i.e., with a focus on "use versus need." What will be revealed (similar to O_2 therapy) is a practice that easily qualifies as a nonscience.

ANEMIA

About 90% of RBC transfusions are given to alleviate anemia in nonbleeding patients (2). Anemia is defined as a decrease in the O_2 carrying capacity of blood, which is a reflection of the total mass of circulating RBCs. The measurement of this RBC mass involves the use of chromium-tagged RBCs and is rarely performed in clinical practice. Instead, the hemoglobin concentration and hematocrit are used as surrogate measures of the RBC mass. The standard clinical definition of anemia is a hemoglobin <13 g/dL in adult men, and <12 g/dL in adult, nonpregnant women. However, these definitions can be misleading, as explained next.

Hemoglobin and Hematocrit

The hematocrit (Hct) and hemoglobin (Hb) concentration have one major shortcoming as surrogate measures of the RBC mass; i.e., they are influenced by the plasma volume. This influence is demonstrated in Figure 6.1, which shows the postural changes in Hct and plasma volume in a group of healthy adults (3). Note

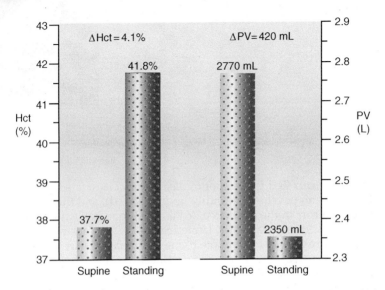

FIGURE 6.1 Postural changes in hematocrit (Hct) and plasma volume (PV) in a group of healthy adults. The numbers above the columns are mean values for each measurement. From Reference 3.

the lower Hct and a higher plasma volume in the supine position. These changes are explained by postural changes in dependent vascular pressures: i.e., when changing from the standing to supine positions, there is a decrease in the capillary hydrostatic pressure in the legs (loss of the gravitational effect), and this promotes the movement of interstitial fluid into the bloodstream. The resulting increase in plasma volume then produces a dilutional decrease in the Hct, even though the RBC mass is unchanged. The change in Hct in Figure 6.1 (4.1%) is equivalent to about one unit of RBCs, so the lower Hct in the supine position could be mistaken for loss of about one unit of blood.

The dilutional effect of an increase in plasma volume will exaggerate the presence and magnitude of anemia, and this can lead to inappropriate RBC transfusions. Conditions associated with increased extracellular (plasma) volume include heart failure, renal failure, aggressive infusion of asanguinous fluids, and a prolonged stay in intensive care units. This latter condition deserves emphasis because ICU patients receive the bulk of RBC transfusions, while clinical studies have shown that the Hct and Hb are unreliable as measures of anemia in this patient population (4,5).

Transfusion Trigger

Despite the confounding influence of plasma volume, the Hb and Hct are the accepted measures for guiding RBC transfusions. Initially, RBC transfusions were recommended when the Hb <10 g/dL or Hct <30% (6), and this "10-30 rule" became the accepted *transfusion trigger* for the next 60 years, until studies aimed at alleviating the transfusion burden discovered that reducing the transfusion threshold to a Hb of 7 g/dL (Hct = 21%) had no adverse consequences, even in critically ill patients and patients with cardiovascular disease (7,8). As a result of these studies, the recommended transfusion trigger has been lowered to Hb <7 g/dL or Hct <21% for most patients (9,10). A slightly higher transfusion trigger (Hb <8 g/dL or Hct <24%) is recommended for patients with cardiovascular disease or undergoing cardiac surgery (9,10), although there is little data to support this recommendation.

Groupthink

Clinicians have been reluctant to adopt the recommendations for a lower transfusion threshold, despite the proven safety of Hb levels down to 7 g/dL. In one survey of transfusion practices in 59 ICUs in the United States (11), 73% of the RBC transfusions were given when the baseline Hb was higher than 7 g/dL. Furthermore, educational initiatives did not improve the transfusion practices in many medical centers. This reluctance to change is a form of "groupthink"; i.e., a condition where individuals make faulty decisions in deference to the traditions of a larger group. There are numerous examples of groupthink in clinical practice, and one of them (i.e., practices related to oxygen) provided the impetus for this book.

Tolerance to Severe Anemia

It is important to emphasize that the recommended transfusion threshold (i.e., Hb = 7 g/dL or Hct = 21%) is not the threshold for the onset of anaerobic metabolism, but is merely the lowest Hb and Hct that have been studied in clinical trials. The point at which anemia compromises aerobic metabolism has been studied in animals, and the results of one of these studies is shown in Figure 6.2 (12). The graph in this figure shows the effects of progressive isovolemic anemia (where blood is withdrawn and replaced by asanguinous fluids) on three measures of systemic oxygenation: the rate of O_2 delivery in arterial blood (DO_2), the percent desaturation of Hb in capillary blood (O_2 extraction), and the whole-body O_2 consumption (VO_2). The influence of progressive anemia on these variables can be explained using the following equation:

$$VO_2 = DO_2 \times O_2 \text{ Extraction} \qquad (6.1)$$

(The relationships in this equation are described in Chapter 2 and are illustrated in Figure 2.2.) As shown in Figure 6.2, the progressive decrease in Hct is accompanied by a steady decrease in DO_2. However, there is also a steady increase in O_2 extraction, and the reciprocal changes in DO_2 and O_2 extraction help to maintain a constant VO_2. When the Hct falls below 10%, the increase in O_2 extraction is no longer able to match the decrease in DO_2, and the VO_2 begins to fall (indicating the onset of aerobic metabolism). Therefore, the study results in Figure 6.2 indicate that anemia will not compromise aerobic metabolism until the Hct falls below 10% (which is equivalent to a Hb < 3.5 g/dL).

Other studies of progressive isovolemic anemia in animals have reported results similar to those in Figure 6.2 (13,14), including a study of animals who were awake and breathing room air (13). Studies of isovolemic anemia in healthy adults have shown that aerobic metabolism is not compromised at a Hb of 5 g/dL (equivalent to a Hct of 15%) (15), but more severe degrees of anemia have not been studied in humans.

Jehovah's Witnesses

The ability of humans to tolerate severe anemia can be inferred from studies of Jehovah's Witness (JW) patients, who refuse blood transfusions on religious grounds. (This refusal is based on a statement in the Bible [Leviticus 17:12], in which God instructs Moses that *"None of you may eat blood, nor may an alien living among you eat blood"*). In one large study of 322 JW patients who underwent cardiac surgery (where about half of the patients normally receive RBC transfusions), the JW patients had fewer postoperative complications (including myocardial infarctions), a shorter length of stay in hospital, and a lower mortality rate, when compared to patients who received RBC transfusions (16). Although the Hct and Hb levels were not reported, this study demonstrates that humans can tolerate more severe degrees of anemia than are normally allowed. (*Note:* The adverse impact of RBC transfusions on outcomes in this study is explained by the numerous complications of RBC transfusions, which are beyond the scope of this chapter.)

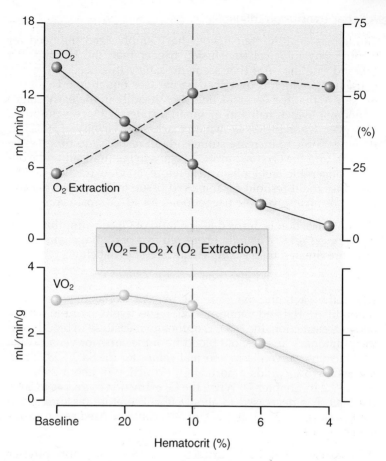

FIGURE 6.2 The influence of progressive isovolemic anemia on O_2 delivery (DO_2), O_2 extraction, and O_2 consumption (VO_2) in primates. The dotted red line indicates the threshold Hct for the onset of anaerobic metabolism. Data from Reference 12.

Summary

The information just presented shows that aerobic metabolism is not compromised until the Hb and Hct fall to levels that are below the levels that trigger RBC transfusions. This means that RBC transfusions are NOT based on tissue O_2 needs, but are based on Hb and Hct levels. The ability to tolerate severe anemia explains why "anemic shock" is not a clinical entity.

A Better Transfusion Trigger

Guidelines on RBC transfusions have emphasized the need for a more physiological transfusion trigger than the Hb and Hct (9), and one measure that seems to satisfy this need is the "O_2 extraction," which is described earlier (see Equation 6.1). Figure 6.2 shows that the O_2 extraction rises steadily in the early stages of anemia, which helps to maintain a constant O_2 consumption. However, when the O_2 extraction reaches the vicinity of 50%, it is no longer able to increase sufficiently in response to progressive anemia, and the O_2 consumption begins to fall (indicating the onset of anaerobic metabolism). Therefore, an O_2 extraction of 50% identifies the threshold for impaired tissue oxygenation (12) and would be an appropriate trigger point for RBC transfusions.

The O_2 extraction is derived as the ratio of O_2 consumption to O_2 delivery (VO_2/DO_2, usually expressed as a percentage), but it can be approximated by the simple equation shown below:

$$O_2 \text{ Extraction} = SaO_2 - SvO_2 \qquad (6.2)$$

where the SaO_2 and SvO_2 are the percent oxyhemoglobin saturation in arterial and venous blood, respectively. (For the whole-body O_2 extraction, the SvO_2 is optimally measured in blood from the pulmonary arteries, but blood from the superior vena cava is a viable alternative.) Using normal values for the SaO_2 (98%) and the SvO_2 (75%) yields a normal O_2 extraction of about 25% (see Figure 2.2 in Chapter 2). When the O_2 extraction increases to 50%, the SvO_2 has decreased to about 50%. Therefore (assuming the SaO_2 is close to 100%), an SvO_2 of 50% could be used as a transfusion trigger (17).

It seems clear that the O_2 extraction and SvO_2 are more physiological transfusion triggers than the Hb or Hct, yet there has been little interest in adopting these measures. One possible reason for this reluctance is the need for a central venous catheter to sample blood from the superior vena cava. Another more likely reason is an adamantine obeisance to tradition.

RESPONSE TO RBC TRANSFUSIONS

The last section demonstrated that most RBC transfusions are given when tissue oxygenation is not compromised, so it is not unreasonable to assume that most RBC transfusions will not enhance tissue oxygenation further (which would promote hypermetabolism). However, there is more to the RBC transfusion story (see next).

Table 6.1 Relationship Between Hematocrit and Blood Viscosity

Hematocrit (%)	Relative Viscosity (water = 1)	Absolute Viscosity (centipoise)
0	1.4	—
10	1.8	1.2
20	2.1	1.5
30	2.8	1.8
40	3.7	2.3
50	4.8	2.9
60	5.8	3.8

From Reference 20.

Blood Viscosity

Blood has a built-in feature that resists blood flow. This feature is the *viscosity,* which is defined as the resistance of a fluid to a change in flow rate (18). It is also described as the "gooiness" of a fluid (19). The viscosity of blood is the result of cross-linking of RBCs by fibrinogen (evident as rouleaux formation), and the concentration of RBCs (the hematocrit, or Hct) is the principal determinant of blood viscosity. The influence of Hct on blood viscosity is shown in Table 6.1 (20). Note that blood viscosity can be expressed in absolute or relative terms (relative to water). The viscosity of plasma (Hct = 0) is only slightly higher than that of water, while the viscosity of whole blood at a normal Hct of 45% is about 3 times greater than plasma and about 4 times greater than water. Erythrocytes are stored in concentrates (packed RBCs) that have a Hct of about 60% and are excessively "gooey." The influence of Hct on blood viscosity is the single most important factor that determines the hemodynamic effect of RBC transfusions.

Non-Newtonian Fluids

The viscosity of some fluids varies inversely with the velocity of flow (18). These fluids are called *non-Newtonian* fluids, and blood is one of them. (Another one is ketchup, which is thick and sluggish when you begin to pour it, but once it starts to flow, it thins out and flows more easily.) The non-Newtonian behavior of blood provides a defense against vascular injury; i.e., blood flow in the area of a punctured blood vessel will decrease (e.g., from external compression due to hematoma formation), and this increases blood viscosity, causing a further reduction in blood flow, and so on. This process helps to limit blood loss from the punctured vessel, while the thickened blood helps to seal the vessel. However, this behavior also magnifies the negative influence of blood viscosity on peripheral blood flow (see next).

Flow Resistance

The influence of viscosity on peripheral blood flow is described by the Hagen-Poiseuille equation (shown below), which identifies the determinants of flow through small tubes (21).

$$Q = \Delta P \times (\pi\, r^4 / 8\, \mu L) \qquad (6.3)$$

According to this equation, flow (Q) through a small tube is directly related to the pressure gradient along the tube (ΔP) and the fourth power of the radius (r) of the tube and is inversely related to the length (L) of the tube and the viscosity (μ) of the fluid.

The final term in the equation is the reciprocal of resistance (1/R), so flow resistance can be described as:

$$R = 8\, \mu L / \pi\, r^4 \qquad (6.4)$$

Resistance to flow is thus directly related to blood viscosity, and the effect is magnified by a factor of eight.

Cardiac Output

Figure 6.3 shows the influence of a progressive increase in Hb concentration on the systemic vascular resistance and cardiac output in healthy adults (15). In this case, a twofold increase in Hb (from 6 to 12 g/dL) is accompanied by a proportional increase in systemic vascular resistance and a similar (almost 50%) reduction in cardiac output. This reduction in cardiac output will limit the ability of RBC transfusions to enhance systemic O_2 delivery (DO_2), as shown by the following equation:

$$DO_2 = CO \times (1.34 \times [Hb] \times SaO_2) \qquad (6.5)$$

where CO is cardiac output, and the variables in parentheses are the determinants of the arterial O_2 content: 1.34 is the O_2 carrying capacity of Hb, [Hb] is the hemoglobin concentration, and SaO_2 is the fractional oxyhemoglobin saturation in arterial blood. Thus, when RBC transfusions increase the Hb concentration, the concomitant decrease in cardiac output limits or cancels the effect on O_2 delivery.

Protective Countermeasures

By reducing blood flow, the viscosity effect of RBC transfusions can be viewed as a countermeasure that helps to protect the tissues from excessive exposure to oxygen and the associated risk of oxidative cell injury. Another countermeasure with similar intent is the vasoconstrictor response to inhaled O_2, which is described in Chapter 5.

Tissue Oxygenation

The influence of RBC transfusions on tissue oxygenation is demonstrated in Figure 6.4, using the systemic O_2 consumption to evaluate the adequacy of tissue oxygenation. The data in this graph are from a group of postoperative patients with severe nor-

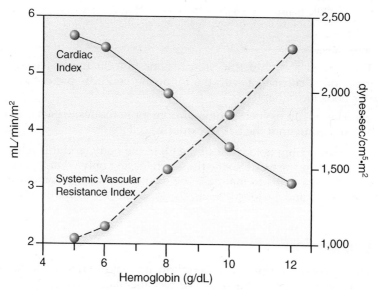

FIGURE 6.3 The effect of a progressive rise in hemoglobin concentration on the size-adjusted cardiac output and systemic vascular resistance in healthy adults. Data from Reference 15.

movolemic anemia (Hb <7 g/dL) who were transfused to raise the Hb above 7 g/dL. As indicated, the RBC transfusions increased the (mean) Hb level from 6.1 to 8 g/dL (a 32% increase), but the O_2 consumption remained unchanged, indicating that the RBC transfusions did not enhance tissue oxygenation in these patients. Note that the pretransfusion O_2 consumption was within the normal range (represented by the vertical bar on the right), indicating that tissue oxygenation was not compromised when the RBCs were transfused. In this situation, RBC transfusions are not expected to further increase tissue O_2 levels.

The response in Figure 6.4 has been reported in several other studies (see the review in Reference 22), indicating that *when aerobic metabolism is not compromised, RBC transfusions do not enhance tissue oxygenation*. Since most RBC transfusions are given when aerobic metabolism is not compromised (as demonstrated in the first section of the chapter), it is possible to conclude that most RBC transfusions do not enhance tissue oxygenation. This is supported in the following statement from a clinical practice guideline on RBC transfusions in critically ill patients (23):

> "RBC transfusion should not be considered an absolute method to improve tissue oxygenation in critically ill patients."

Implications

The limited ability of RBC transfusions to influence tissue oxygenation is consistent with the following concepts presented in this book (see Chapter 3).

1. There is an oxygen-poor environment in tissues, which is designed to limit the risk of oxidative cell injury.

2. Hemoglobin holds 98% of the O_2 in the body, and it is reluctant to release O_2 into the tissues, releasing only what is needed. This helps to maintain the oxygen-poor environment in tissues and thereby protect the tissues from oxidative damage.

SUMMATION

This chapter has identified the following major flaws in the current use of RBC transfusions to correct anemia:

1. The hemoglobin and hematocrit are inadequate as measures of anemia (and as transfusion triggers) because they are influenced by the plasma volume, which is often abnormal in the type of patients who receive RBC transfusions.

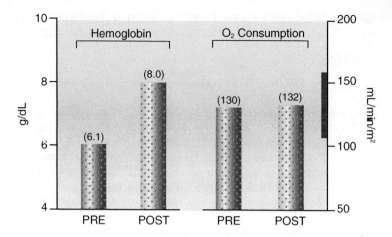

FIGURE 6.4 Influence of RBC transfusions on hemoglobin (Hb) concentration and systemic O_2 consumption in 11 postoperative patients with severe normovolemic anemia (Hb <7 g/dL). The normal range for O_2 consumption is indicated by the vertical bar on the right. Numbers in parentheses represent mean values. Data from personal observations.

2. The "O_2 extraction" is superior to the Hb or Hct as a transfusion trigger because it can detect when tissue oxygenation is threatened or impaired. However, it is rarely used.

3. Aerobic metabolism is not compromised until the Hb falls below 3 g/dL, yet the transfusion of RBCs typically occurs when the Hb falls below 7 or 8 g/dL. This means that RBC transfusions are usually given when aerobic metabolism is not compromised.

4. The viscosity effect of RBC transfusions reduces cardiac output, and this limits the influence of RBC transfusions on systemic O_2 delivery. This means that a transfusion-related increase in hemoglobin or hematocrit does not ensure an increase in oxygen delivery.

5. When aerobic metabolism is not compromised, RBC transfusions do not enhance tissue oxygenation. The reluctance of hemoglobin (Hb) to release O_2 into the tissues, unless it is needed, is a protective device that limits the risk of oxidative tissue injury.

Considered individually or together, these flaws provide convincing evidence that RBC transfusions are NOT based on tissue

O_2 needs. In fact, they are not based on anything that has scientific merit.

REFERENCES

1. From the American Red Cross website (americanredcross.org), accessed on 2/15/2021.
2. Corwin HL, Gettinger A, Pearl R, et al. The CRIT study: anemia and blood transfusion in the critically ill – Current clinical practice in the United States. Crit Care Med 2004; 32:39-52.
3. Jacob G, Raj SR, Ketch T, et al. Postural pseudoanemia: posture-dependent change in hematocrit. Mayo Clin Proc 2005; 80:611-614.
4. Jones JG, Holland BM, Wardrop CAJ. Total circulating red cells versus hematocrit as a primary descriptor of oxygen transport by the blood. Br J Hematol 1990;76:228–232.
5. Cordts PR, LaMorte WW, Fisher JB, et al. Poor predictive value of hematocrit and hemodynamic parameters for erythrocyte deficits after extensive elective vascular operations. Surg Gynecol Obstet 1992;175:243–248.
6. Adam RC, Lundy JS. Anesthesia in cases of poor risk: Some suggestions for decreasing the risk. Surg Gynecol Obstet 1942: 74:1011-1101.
7. Hebert PC, Wells G, Blajchman MA, et al. A multicenter, randomized, controlled clinical trial of transfusion requirements in critical care. N Engl J Med 1999; 340:409-417.
8. Hebert PC, Yetisir E, Martin C, et al. Is a low transfusion threshold safe in critically ill patients with cardiovascular disease? Crit Care Med 2001; 29:227-234.
9. Carson JL, Guyatt G, Heddle NM, et al. Clinical practice guidelines from the AABB: Red blood cell transfusion threshold and storage. JAMA 2016; 316: 2025-2035.
10. Mueller M, van Remoortel H, Meybohm P, et al. Patient blood management: Recommendations from the 2018 Frankfurt Consensus Conference. JAMA 2019; 321:983-997.
11. Seitz KP, Sevransky JE, Martin GS, et al. Evaluation of RBC transfusion practice in adult ICUs and the effect of restrictive transfusion protocols on routine care. Crit Care Med 2017; 45:271-281.
12. Wilkerson DK, Rosen AL, Gould SA, et al. Oxygen extraction ratio: a valid indicator of myocardial metabolism in anemia. J Surg Res 1987;42:629–634.
13. Nielses VG, Baird MS, Brix AE, Matalon S. Extreme progressive isovolemic hemodilution with 5% albumin, PentaLyte, or Hextend does not cause hepatic ischemic or histologic injury in rabbits. Anesthesiol 1999; 90:1428-1440.

14. Wilkerson DK, Rosen AL, Sehgal LR, et al. Limits of cardiac compensation in anemic baboons. Surgery 1988; 103:665-670.
15. Weiskopf RB, Viele M, Feiner J, et al. Human cardiovascular and metabolic response to acute, severe, isovolemic anemia. JAMA 1998; 279:217-221.
16. Pattakos G, Koch CG, Brizzio ME, et al. Outcome of patients who refuse transfusion after cardiac surgery. Arch Intern Med 2012; 172:1154-1160.
17. Vallet B, Robin E, Lebutte G. Venous oxygen saturation as a transfusion trigger. Crit Care 2010; 14:213.
18. Baskurt OK, Meiselman HJ. Blood rheology and hemodynamics. Semin Thromb Hemost 2003; 29:435-450.
19. Vogel S. Life in Moving Fluids. Princeton: Princeton University Press, 1981: 11-24.
20. Documenta Geigy Scientific Tables. 7th ed. Basel: Documenta Geigy, 1966:557-558.
21. Chien S, Usami S, Skalak R. Blood flow in small tubes. In Renkin EM, Michel CC (eds). Handbook of Physiology. Section 2: The cardiovascular system. Volume IV. The microcirculation. Bethesda: American Physiological Society,1984:217-249.
22. Nielsen ND, Martin-Loeches I, Wentowski C. The effects of red blood cell transfusions on tissue oxygenation and the microcirculation in the intensive care unit: A systematic review. Transf Med Rev 2017; 31:205-222.
23. Napolitano LM, Kurek S, Luchette FA, et al. Clinical practice guideline: Red blood cell transfusion in adult trauma and critical care. Crit Care Med 2009; 37:3124-3157.

How Destructive is Oxygen?

What is oxidation?

7

"I brought fire into your midst, and it consumed you, and reduced you to ashes."

Ezekiel 28:17

Have you ever wondered why food is stored in vacuum-sealed containers, or why we use cellophane wrapping and tightly sealed plastic containers to keep food "fresh"? The guiding principle in all these measures is to avoid exposure to air, or more specifically, to oxygen in the air, because oxygen promotes the decomposition of organic matter. Oxygen has the unique ability to disrupt the carbon bonds that hold organic molecules together, and this results in the breakdown or degradation of the molecules. This breakdown releases energy, and if the molecule is a high-energy substrate (an organic fuel), the energy released can be enough to power machines or living organisms. The dual actions of oxygen to destroy organic matter and release life-giving energy makes oxygen a source both of life *and* death. The disruptive actions of oxygen are the result of a chemical reaction known as *oxidation*; a reaction that provides the foundation for oxygen's role in the aerobic world.

THE CHEMISTRY OF OXIDATION

The French chemist extraordinaire, Antoine Lavoisier, is credited with the discovery of a gas he named "oxygene" (although he was not the first to isolate this gas). He also introduced the term "oxidation" to describe a chemical reaction in which oxygen is added to another reactant to produce an oxide. The opposite effect, the removal of oxygen, which reduces an oxide to its original state, was called a "reduction" reaction. The chemistry of oxidation reactions is based on the electron configuration of the oxygen molecule, which is described next.

The Oxygen Molecule

Oxygen in its natural or ground state is a diatomic molecule (O_2) with a covalent double bond linking the two oxygen atoms. It has

16 electrons (8 from each atom) that are arranged in the config-uration shown in Figure 7.1 (1). In the quantum atom, electrons occupy energy domains known as *orbitals* (indicated by the circles in Figure 7.1), and each orbital can accept a pair of electrons that spin in opposite directions (indicated by the arrows). These orbit-als are arranged in concentric shells of increasing energy as they move away from the nucleus. As electrons are added, they fill the orbitals in the lowest energy shells first (i.e., the ones closest to the nucleus) before moving up to the next level. Note that the outer-most orbitals are not filled, and the O_2 molecule can accept four electrons to completely fill its orbitals.

Spin Restriction

The unpaired electrons in the O_2 molecule is a characteristic fea-ture of *free radicals*, which are *atoms or molecules that have one or more unpaired electrons, and are capable of an independent existence* (hence the term "free") (1). Free radicals tend to be highly reac-tive, as a consequence of their unfilled atomic orbitals. However, the O_2 molecule does not adhere to this behavior and is sluggish-ly reactive, despite being a free radical. This is explained by the outermost electrons in the O_2 molecule, which have the same di-rectional spin. One of the quantum rules for the atom is that two electrons cannot occupy the same orbital if they have the same directional spin. (This is the Pauli Exclusion Principle, named af-ter the puckish Austrian physicist, Wolfgang Pauli.) This means that oxygen cannot accept an electron pair, because this would result in two electrons with the same directional spin occupying the same orbital, which is a quantum impossibility. As a result, the O_2 molecule can accept only one electron for each oxidation reaction, and this *spin restriction* hampers the reactivity of oxygen. It also has a profound influence on the metabolism of O_2 in mito-chondria, which is described in Chapter 8.

Redox Reactions

Chemical reactions involving O_2 are characterized by a transfer of electrons to the O_2 molecule (to fill its outer atomic orbitals). The loss of electrons in the donor molecule is known as *oxidation* (replacing Lavoisier's definition), and is accompanied by loss of hydrogen ions or "dehydrogenation." Conversely, the gain in electrons by O_2 (or any chemical species that accepts electrons) is known as *reduction*. Since oxidation is always accompanied by reduction, the overall reaction is known as a *redox reaction*.

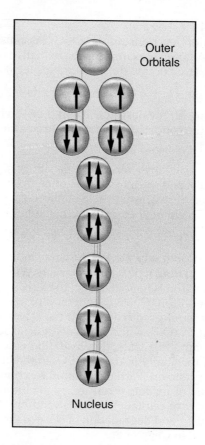

FIGURE 7.1 Orbital diagram showing the configuration of electrons in the oxygen molecule (O_2). Circles represent atomic orbitals, and the arrows show the directional spin of the electrons that occupy each orbital. The configuration of the outermost electrons restricts the reactivity of oxygen. See text for explanation. Adapted from Reference 1.

The oxidation of an organic molecule results in loss of electrons from the carbon bonds that hold the molecule together. This cleaves the carbon bonds, and the result can be complete breakdown of the substrate (complete oxidation), or disruption of a specific site on the molecule (partial oxidation). Each type of oxidation reaction has different consequences, as explained next.

Complete Oxidation

Complete oxidation reactions result in total dissolution of the organic substrate. A familiar example is the oxidative breakdown of glucose ($C_6H_{12}O_6$) that occurs during aerobic metabolism.

$$C_6H_{12}O_6 + 6\,O_2 \rightarrow 6\,CO_2 + 6\,H_2O \qquad (7.1)$$

These reactions are highly destructive, but they can be a source of usable energy if the conditions are favorable (see later).

Partial Oxidation

Partial oxidation reactions alter a specific site or segment of the substrate molecule, and the alteration is often deleterious. An example of this type of reaction is the oxidation of oxyhemoglobin (heme-Fe^{2+}-O_2) to form methemoglobin (heme-Fe^{3+}):

$$(\text{heme-Fe}^2\text{-O}_2) - e^- \rightarrow (\text{heme-Fe}^{3+}) + O_2^{\cdot} \qquad (7.2)$$

The iron in hemoglobin is located in the heme moiety and is present as ferrous (Fe^{2+}) iron, which binds oxygen. When hemoglobin is oxidized, an electron is removed from the ferrous iron, converting it to ferric (Fe^{3+}) iron, which cannot bind oxygen. In addition, the electron that is released reacts with the released O_2 to form the *superoxide radical* ($O_2^{\cdot}$), which can have several adverse effects (described in Chapter 8). Thus, this oxidation reaction not only results in loss of the ability to transport O_2 in the bloodstream, it also produces a cytotoxin. Partial oxidation reactions are responsible for all forms of oxidative cell injury, including loss of the functional integrity of cell membranes, strand breakage in DNA and RNA molecules, and degradation of cell proteins. These reactions are described in Chapter 8.

OXIDATION AS A SOURCE OF ENERGY

The energy that powers our lives comes from the sun, and how this energy is made available to us is illustrated in Figure 7.2.

Photosynthesis

The first step in providing energy for this planet is carried out by photosynthesis, which captures the radiant energy in sunlight and transforms it into chemical energy that is stored in carbohydrate molecules. Building a carbohydrate molecule (basic formula CH_2O) requires a source of carbon, hydrogen, and oxygen, with the hydrogen requirement being double that of the other constituents. To obtain the needed hydrogen, photosynthesis uses the energy in sunlight to disrupt water molecules (H_2O), and one of the byproducts of this action is the release of O_2 into the atmosphere. The carbon and oxygen atoms are supplied by CO_2 in the atmosphere. (The mechanisms involved in photosynthesis are complex and are beyond the scope of this presentation.) The overall reaction for photosynthesis is shown in Figure 7.2, using dextrose as the carbohydrate. (Photosynthesis produces simple sugars or monosaccharides, and dextrose is the most common end product.) Note that photosynthesis not only introduces energy into the organic world, it also provides a means for accessing this energy by producing oxygen.

Combustion Reactions

The available energy in the carbohydrate molecules (and in all organic molecules) is stored in the carbon bonds that hold the molecules together, and oxygen (oxidation) has the unique ability to break these bonds and release the energy. The energy released by oxidation is transformed from chemical energy to thermal energy or heat. These heat-producing or *exothermic* reactions are called *combustion reactions*. When complete, these reactions break down the organic substrate into CO_2 and H_2O, and this allows the energy cycle in Figure 7.2 to continue.

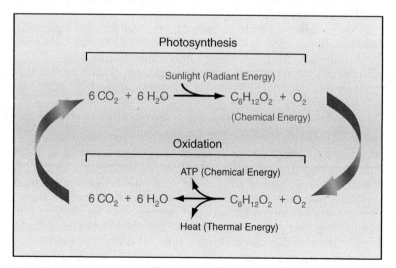

FIGURE 7.2 The energy cycle for all living organisms. Photosynthesis captures the radiant energy in sunlight and transforms it into chemical energy, and oxidation releases the chemical energy so it can be used to perform the work of living.

The energy yield from combustion reactions is influenced by the rate of the reaction; i.e., faster reactions produce more complete oxidations, and this increases the energy yield. Oxygen is a relatively sluggish oxidant (because of the electron spin restriction mentioned earlier), and an accelerant is needed to optimize the energy yield. Combustion reactions are temperature sensitive, and high temperatures are used to accelerate these reactions in mechanical engines. The major accelerants for oxidative metabolism are oxidase and dehydrogenase enzymes.

Organic Fuels

The strength of carbon bonds is not uniform (e.g., double bonds are stronger than single bonds), and stronger bonds release more energy when disrupted. Organic molecules that are endowed with high-energy bonds serve as *organic fuels*. (A fuel is defined as any substance that generates heat when oxidized, but the term is used here to denote a substance that generates useful heat.) The principal organic fuels are listed below.

1. *Fossil fuels* are derived from decomposed organic matter that has been buried for centuries. These fuels include petroleum products (e.g., gasoline, heating oil), coal, and natural gas. Together, these fuels account for 80% of the energy use in the United States (2).
2. *Nutrient fuels* include carbohydrates, proteins, and lipids. Although not included in traditional lists of organic fuels, they are the sole source of energy in aerobic life-forms.
3. *Biofuels* are renewable fuels derived from organic matter that has not decayed. Ethanol is the original, and most widely used, biofuel.
4. *Wood* is a low-carbon fuel that accounts for only about 2% of the energy use in the United States (2).

The energy content of the major organic fuels is shown in Table 7.1. Note that lipids have the third highest energy content of all the organic fuels; greater than coal, and only 2.4 kcal/g less than gasoline. Vegetable oils have been an alternative fuel for diesel engines since Rudolph Diesel used peanut oil in his early engine designs (3), and today vegetable oils are used as biodiesel fuels. Lipids are also the major storage form of energy in the human body. The average-sized adult has about 165,000 kcal of stored energy: adipose tissue contributes 141,000 kcal (85%), muscle proteins contribute 24,000 kcal (14.5%), and glycogen contributes 900 kcal (0.5%) (4).

Table 7.1 Energy Yield from the Oxidation of Organic Fuels

Organic Fuel	Energy Yield*	
Natural Gas	54 kJ/g	12.9 kcal/g
Gasoline	48 kJ/g	11.5 kcal/g
Lipids	38 kJ/g	9.1 kcal/g
Coal	34 kJ/g	8.1 kcal/g
Ethanol	30 kJ/g	7.2 kcal/g
Charcoal	23kJ/g	5.5 kcal/g
Wood	20 kJ/g	4.8 kcal/g
Protein	17 kJ/g	4.0 kcal/g
Carbohydrates	16 kJ/g	3.7 kcal/g

*kJ = kilojoules, kcal = kilocalories. Conversions: kJ/g x 0.239 = kcal/g, kcal/g x 4.2 = kJ/g.
From the Transportation Energy Data Book . Available at www.tedb.ornl.gov (Accessed 2/28/2021).

Carbon Dioxide

All combustion reactions produce CO_2, which can be problematic. The primacy of CO_2 removal in the human body is emphasized in the first two chapters of this book, and the consequences of CO_2 accumulation in the atmosphere have been a major concern (to some) for several years. In the United States (a major contributor to the rise in atmospheric CO_2), the combustion of fossil fuels accounts for 93% of the anthropogenic CO_2 emissions, and 50% of this is from petroleum products (5). Of interest in this regard is a comparison of combustion reactions for octane (a major ingredient in gasoline) and methane (the principal component of natural gas). Octane is a hydrocarbon with an eight-carbon backbone (C_8H_{18}), and the combustion reaction is as follows:

$$2\ C_8H_{18} + 25\ O_2 \rightarrow 16\ CO_2 + 18\ H_2O \qquad (7.3)$$

Methane is the smallest hydrocarbon, with a single carbon atom (CH_4), and the combustion reaction is:

$$CH_4 + 2\,O_2 \rightarrow CO_2 + 2\,H_2O \qquad (7.4)$$

The combustion of natural gas generates much less CO_2 than the combustion of petroleum products, and natural gas also has the highest energy content of the organic fuels. Thus, a transition to natural gas will help to slow the rise in atmospheric CO_2. However, the real solution to the atmospheric CO_2 problem is to transition away from fossil fuels altogether.

Aerobic Metabolism

Antoine Lavoisier was the first to recognize the similarities between aerobic metabolism and combustion, and stated: "Respiration is thus a process of combustion, in truth very slow, but exactly like that of charcoal" (6). The comparisons in Table 7.2 show that aerobic metabolism is essentially a biochemical version of an automobile engine. Both use an organic fuel mixed with O_2, and use accelerant techniques to optimize the energy yield. They both generate heat and produce CO_2 as an end product. Finally, both

Table 7.2	Internal Combustion Engines	
	Automobile Engine	**Aerobic Metabolism**
Type of Engine	Mechanical	Biochemical
Type of Fuel	Fossil Fuel	Nutrient Fuel
Ignition	Spark	Always On
Accelerants	High Temp., High O_2	Enzymes
Energy Release	Heat	Heat
Transducer	Piston	ATP
Major Waste Product	CO_2	CO_2
Energy Efficiency	20%	35%

engines have a transduction mechanism that allows the thermal energy to perform work, but neither does this very well, as indicated by the poor energy efficiency.

Energy Utilization

Energy efficiency is a measure of the fraction of available energy that is used to perform work. The energy efficiency of gasoline engines is notoriously poor (on average about 20%), and even the sophisticated engines in Formula 1 racing cars are unable to achieve energy efficiencies above 40%. The same limitation applies to aerobic metabolism. The energy efficiency of 35% in Table 7.2 was obtained by comparing the energy yield from glucose oxidation ex vivo with the energy yield from the ATP molecules produced by glucose metabolism. This is demonstrated in the steps below.

1. The energy yield from the oxidation of organic fuels (called the "heat of combustion") is measured under controlled conditions in a sealed chamber called a "bomb calorimeter." When glucose is oxidized in this manner, the heat of combustion is 673 kcal per mole (7). One mole of glucose is 180 grams, so 673 kcal/mol is equivalent to 3.7 kcal/gram, which is the energy yield from carbohydrates in Table 7.1.

2. Glucose metabolism produces 32 ATP molecules, and the energy yield from ATP hydrolysis is 7.3 kcal/mole (8), so the yield of usable energy from glucose metabolism is 7.3 x 32 = 234 kcal/mole.

3. The energy efficiency of glucose metabolism is thus: 234/673 x 100 = 35%.

The inefficiency of energy utilization, both inside and outside the body, indicates that oxidative breakdown of organic matter is excessive for the yield of usable energy. This shines a light on the destructive nature of oxidation, which is the focus of the next section.

OXIDATIVE DESTRUCTION

Oxidation can generate usable energy when the following conditions are present: there is an energy-rich substrate that is completely oxidized, the reaction is accelerated (e.g., by enzymes), and there is a transduction system to convert the thermal energy into a more suitable form for performing work (e.g., ATP production). However, most oxidation reactions do not have the necessary conditions for releasing usable energy, but instead serve only to damage or destroy organic matter. This section focuses on these reactions.

Autoxidation

Oxidation reactions that occur spontaneously are known as au-to-oxidations, usually shortened to *autoxidation* (9). These reactions are the result of exposure to atmospheric O_2 at ambient temperatures, and examples include the degradation of food products and cooking oils, the decomposition of animal and human carcasses, and the degradation of rubber and select plastic polymers (e.g., nylon). The heat produced by these reactions is imperceptible, and the principal result is gradual degradation of the oxidized material. Autoxidation is a slow but relentless march to destruction, and continues as long as there is available substrate.

Oxidation of Lipids

The lipids in food products and vegetable oils are prone to oxidation, as are the lipids in our cell membranes.

Dietary Lipids

The oxidation of dietary lipids occurs most readily in polyunsaturated fatty acids (PUFAs). These lipids are susceptible to oxidative disruption because they have multiple carbon-carbon double bonds (a characteristic feature), which rupture more easily than single bonds (7). (The term "unsaturated" refers to the reduced hydrogen content of lipid molecules with carbon-carbon double bonds, because these bonds bind less hydrogen than single bonds. "Polyunsaturated" indicates the presence of more than one double bond.) PUFAs are essential fatty acids and must be obtained from the diet. The principal sources are fish, fish oils, nuts, and vegetable oils (10). The oxidation of these lipids produces an unpleasant odor and foul taste; a condition known as *rancidity* (10,11). Oxidized PUFAs can be toxic if ingested (12), but the disagreeable odor and taste of rancid food is a detriment to ingestion. As a result, the oxidation of dietary lipids has little or no pathological impact and serves only as a source of food spoilage. However, the oxidation of lipids in our cell membranes can be a source of pathological, and even life-threatening, damage, as explained next.

Membrane Lipids

The lipophilic interior of cell membranes is rich in PUFAs, which are essential for maintaining the fluidity of cell membranes because of their low melting point. The oxidation of membrane lipids is described in detail in the next chapter, and is only briefly summarized here. The oxidation of PUFAs in cell membranes is usually triggered by reactive oxygen species or free iron, and the oxidation continues as self-regenerating or chain reaction that propagates along the cell membrane (13). As the PUFAs oxidize, they polymerize and lose their fluidity, causing the cell membrane to become stiff and leaky. The selective transport functions of the cell membrane are then lost, which is a prelude to cell death. The damage from this process can be curtailed by α-tocopherol (vitamin E), which is present in cell membranes, and blocks the propagation of the chain reaction. (See Chapter 12 for more on vitamin E.)

Drying Oils

PUFA-rich oils are added to paints, stains, and lacquers because their low melting point promotes fluidity (i.e., eases application), while exposure to air oxidizes PUFAs and reduces fluidity (i.e., promotes drying). These oils are called *drying oils*, and the most popular one is linseed oil (also called flaxseed oil).

The problem with drying oils is the risk of *spontaneous combustion*, which can occur in rags soaked with linseed oil and left in an enclosed space. This is a reported cause of fires, one of which destroyed a 38-story office building in Philadelphia PA, and caused the death of three firefighters (14). These fires are attributed to the heat produced by oxidation in the oil-soaked cloth, which causes a rapid rise in temperature in the small spaces of the crumpled cloth, eventually igniting the cloth (15). Although this phenomenon is uncommon, it demonstrates the destructive power of oxidation.

The Oxygen Holocaust

The Earth was formed about 4.5 billion years ago, and the early atmosphere was a product of volcanic eruptions, consisting mainly of water vapor, CO_2, and sulfurous gases. Oxygenation of the atmosphere began about 2.5 billion years ago, thanks to the proliferation of photosynthetic microbes known as cyanobacteria. Atmospheric O_2 levels initially rose to about half the current level (0.1 atm or 10%), and then stayed steady until 500 million years ago, when there was a second spike in atmospheric O_2 that reached the current level (0.21 atm or 21%) (16).

The rise in atmospheric O_2 is known as the *Great Oxidation Event* (17), but it has also been called *the Oxygen Holocaust* (18). The latter title is based on the theory that the rise in atmospheric O_2 caused widespread oxidative damage in existing lifeforms, and only those organisms that developed a means of "antioxidant protection" were able to thrive and evolve in the oxygenated atmosphere. According to this scenario, *life is possible on this planet not just because of oxygen, but because of the ability to protect against the destructive effects of oxygen.*

Oxidative Stress

The description of the Oxygen Holocaust is based on the principle that the potential for oxidative destruction is determined by the balance between the intensity of exposure to O_2 and the ability to protect against this exposure. The O_2 threat in vivo is from reactive derivatives of O_2, known as *reactive oxygen species* (ROS), and protection against the damaging effects of ROS is provided by a diverse group of chemical compounds known as *antioxidants*. *Oxidative stress* occurs when the production of ROS exceeds the capacity for antioxidant protection. This concept is the basis of our current understanding about the pathophysiology of oxidative cell injury. (The actions of ROS are described in Chapter 8, and the protective effects of antioxidants are described in Chapter 12.)

Prematurity

The scenario for the Oxygen Holocaust is not far removed from that of premature infants, who are exposed to atmospheric O_2 before their antioxidant defenses are fully developed. Exposure to O_2 in the fetal lung is negligible because the lung is filled with fluid (and O_2 does not readily dissolve in aqueous fluids, as described in Chapter 3). Antioxidant activity is correspondingly low in the developing lung, and it begins to appear very late in gestation (19). At the moment of birth, the lungs fill with air, and are abruptly exposed to PO_2 levels of 100 mm Hg (or even higher if supplemental O_2 is used). This creates an oxidant stress when the birth (and the antioxidant protection) is premature. Unprotected O_2 exposure has been implicated in a pathological condition known as *bronchopulmonary dysplasia* (20), which often leads to chronic respiratory problems (20). Although less certain, oxidant stress may also play a role in the lung inflammation associated with *neonatal respiratory distress syndrome* (21).

Premature exposure to O_2 is also a causative factor in the *retinopathy of prematurity* (22), which is characterized by disordered development of the retinal blood vessels, and can lead to retinal detachment and blindness. Judicious use of O_2 has decreased the incidence of this disorder.

Oxidative Cell Injury

Partial oxidation reactions threaten the functional integrity of all cell components, and Table 7.3 shows the major types of oxidative

TABLE 7.3	Major Forms of Oxidative Cell Injury
Injury	**Consequences**
Cell Membranes • Oxidation of polyunsaturated fatty acids, which propagates as a chain reaction	• Loss of membrane fluidity • Leaky membranes • Osmotic cell lysis
Nucleic Acids • Modified nucleotide bases • Strand breakage • Telomere shortening	• Cell senescence • Apoptosis • Genetic mutations
Proteins • Degradation of amino acids • Polypeptide disruption, which can propagate as a chain reaction	• Dysfunctional enzymes • Altered cell signaling • Disrupted membrane transport

cell injury and the adverse consequences. Oxidative injury has been implicated in a multitude of diseases, especially those in which inflammation plays a major role. The interest in this condition is demonstrated by the 30,000 articles published yearly on this topic (23). Oxidative cell injury is the focus of the next chapter.

CORROSION

Oxidation is also a prominent source of destruction in the inorganic world, and a brief mention of this seems warranted. A familiar example of this destruction is the corrosion of metals like iron and steel. Iron is readily oxidized to form iron oxide, and when this occurs in the presence of water, the result is hydrated iron oxide (Fe_2O_3-H_2O), better known as *rust*. Steel is an iron alloy that is also susceptible to rust formation. Metals that are resistant to corrosion include gold, silver, and platinum, and the permanence of these metals may explain why they are so highly valued.

Corrosion is the major cause of catastrophic bridge collapses (over 100 worldwide since the year 2000), and it is a constant threat to the structural integrity of high rise buildings, stadiums, gas and oil pipelines, and all forms of transportation. The magnitude of the corrosion problem is shown by *the cost of fighting corrosion*, which is estimated at *$437 billion annually in the United States* (24); a cost that exceeds all other natural disasters combined.

SUMMATION

The available energy in the organic world is stored in the carbon bonds that hold organic molecules together, and oxidation has the unique ability to disrupt these bonds and release the stored energy. The oxidation of organic fuels provides about 85% of the energy needs of everyday living, and it is the sole source of the energy that sustains aerobic life. However, this comes at a cost, because oxidation destroys the organic substrates that provide the energy (as the introductory quote indicates).

Oxidation reactions can generate usable energy only when certain conditions are present (e.g., the substrate is an energy-rich fuel, etc.). However, these conditions are not present for a majority of oxidation reactions, and these reactions serve only to damage or destroy organic matter.

REFERENCES

1. Halliwell B, Gutteridge JMC. Free Radicals in Biology and Medicine. 5th ed, Oxford: Oxford University Press, 2015:1-29.
2. U.S. Energy Information Administration, Monthly Energy Review, April 2020. (Available at www.eia.gov. Accessed 3/19/2021).
3. Diesel R. Introduction. In: Chalkey AP. Diesel Engines for Land and Marine Work. New York: D. van Norstrand Co, 1912:1-8. (Available on Google Books, accessed 12/5/2021).
4. Cahill GF, Jr. Starvation in man. N Engl J Med 1970; 282:668-675.
5. U.S. Energy Information Association. www.eia.gov. Accessed 3/21/2021.
6. Lavoisier A. Memoir on heat. In Fulton JF, Wilson LG, eds. Selected Readings in the History of Physiology. 2nd ed, Springfield: Charles C Thomas, 1966:137.
7. Lehninger AL. Bioenergetics. New York, W.A. Benjamin, Inc, 1965:15.
8. Alberts B, Johnson A, Lewis J, et al., eds. Molecular Biology of the Cell, 6th ed, New York: Garland Science, 2015:774-776.
9. Walling C. Autoxidation. In Foote CS, Valentine JS, Greenberg A, Liebman JF (eds). Active Oxygen in Chemistry. New York: Blackie Academic and Professional, 1995:24-65.
10. Halliwell B, Gutteridge JMC. Free Radicals in Biology and Medicine. 5th ed, Oxford: Oxford University Press, 2015:199-283.

11. Haman N, Romano A, Asaduzzaman M, et al. A microcalorimetry study on the oxidation of linoleic acid and the control of rancidity. Talanta 2017; 164:407-412.

12. Meydani SN, Dinarello CA. Influence of dietary fatty acids on cytokine production and its clinical implications. Nutr Clin Pract 1993; 8:65-72.

13. Shahidi F, Zhong Y. Lipid oxidation and improving the oxidative stability. Chem Soc Rev 2010; 39:4067-4079.

14. Routely JG, Jennings C, Chubb M. Highrise Office Building Fire, One Meridian Plaza, Philadelphia, Pennsylvania. U.S. Fire Administration/Technical Report Series, USFA-TR-049. Emmitsburg, MD: U.S. Fire Administration, February, 1991.

15. Abraham CJ. A solution to spontaneous combustion in linseed oil formulations. Polymer Degrad Stab 1996; 54:157-166.

16. Holland HD. The oxygenation of the atmosphere and oceans. Phil Trans R Soc B, 2006; 361:903-915.

17. Sessions AL, Doughty DM, Welander PV, et al. The continuing puzzle of the Great Oxidation Event. Curr Biol 2009; 19:R567-R574.

18. Margulis L, Sagan D. The oxygen holocaust. In: Microcosmos - Four Billion Years of Microbial Evolution. Berkeley: University of California Press, 1986:99-114.

19. Frank, L, Sosenko IRS. Development of lung antioxidant enzyme system in late gestation: Possible implications for the prematurely born infant. J Pediatr1987; 110:9-14.

20. Principi N, Di Pietro GM, Esposito S. Bronchopulmonary dysplasia: clinical aspects and preventive and therapeutic strategies. J Transl Med 2018; 16:36.

21. Brus F, van Oeveren W, Okken A, Oetomo SB. Number and activation of circulating polymorphonuclear leukocytes and platelets are associated with disease severity in neonatal respiratory distress syndrome. Pediatr 1997; 99:672-680.

22. Kim SJ, Port AD, Swan R, et al. Retinopathy of prematurity: A review of risk factors and their clinical significance. Surv Ophthalmol 2018; 63:6180637.

23. Sies H. Oxidative stress: eustress and distress in redox homeostasis. In Fink G, ed. Stress: physiology, Biochemistry, and Pathology. Handbook of Stress Series, vol. 3. London: Academic Press, 2019:153-163.

24. Waldman J. Rust. The Longest War. New York: Simon & Schuster, 2016:7.

What are reactive oxygen species?

8

> "Great white sharks in the biochemical sea, these short-lived
> but voracious agents oxidize and damage tissue."

Roy Wolford, MD (a)

The natural tendency for oxygen to disrupt organic molecules is enhanced in aerobic cells by the formation of more reactive derivatives of oxygen known as *reactive oxygen species*. These are the "great white sharks in the biochemical sea," in the introductory quote; a description that highlights the destructive power of these enhanced oxidants. This chapter describes the origins and chemical features of reactive oxygen species, and the different mechanisms of oxidative cell injury.

OXYGEN METABOLISM

Oxygen does not participate directly in the metabolic oxidation of nutrient fuels. Instead, oxidation is carried out by a group of dehydrogenase enzymes, and the electrons that are released are picked up by "electron carriers" (e.g., nicotinamide adenine dinucleotides: NAD and NADP) and transported to the inner membrane in mitochondria. The electrons are then passed along via a series of redox reactions involving four protein complexes (the *electron transport chain*), and the associated movement of hydrogen ions across the inner mitochondrial membrane results in the production of high-energy phosphate compounds (adenosine triphosphate, or ATP). Oxygen sits at the end of the electron transport chain (housed in the cytochrome c oxidase complex), and the "spent" electrons are used to reduce oxygen to water (see Figure 4.1); i.e.,

$$O_2 + 4\,e^- + 4\,H^+ \rightarrow 2\,H_2O \tag{8.1}$$

This reaction serves as an "electron sink" that prevents the buildup of electrons and allows continued functioning of the electron transport chain (and the continued production of ATP).

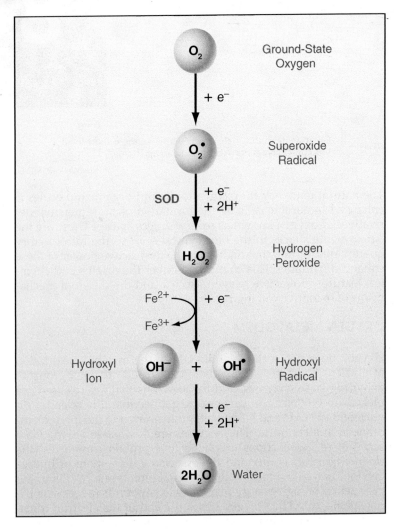

FIGURE 8.1 The reaction sequence for the reduction of oxygen to water, which takes place at the end of the electron transport chain in mitochondria. Free radicals are indicated by a superscripted dot. SOD = superoxide dismutase. See text for explanation.

The four electrons needed to reduce O_2 to water cannot be added in a single reaction because of the electron spin restriction described in the last chapter. As a result, a series of four single-elec-

TABLE 8.1   Reactive Oxygen Species

Free Radicals	Nonradicals
Alkoxyl Radical (LO˙)	Hydrogen Peroxide (H_2O_2)
Hydroxyl Radical (HO˙)	Hypochlorous Acid (HOCL)
Peroxyl Radical (LOO˙)	Lipid Hydroperoxide (LOOH)
Superoxide Radical ($O_2^{˙}$)	Singlet Oxygen ($^1O_2$)

tron reduction reactions is required to reduce O_2 to H_2O, and these are shown in Figure 8.1 (1). This reaction sequence generates three metabolic intermediates: the superoxide radical, hydrogen peroxide, and the hydroxyl radical. These metabolites are more reactive than the parent O_2 molecule, and thus, they are called "reactive oxygen species," commonly abbreviated as ROS. The O_2 metabolites are the not the only ROS; a more complete list is shown in Table 8.1.

Superoxide Radical

The addition of one electron to the O_2 molecule produces the *superoxide radical,* which has one remaining unpaired electron (see Figure 8.2):

$$O_2 + e^- \rightarrow O_2^{˙} \qquad (8.2)$$

(The superscripted dot is the symbol for a *free radical,* which is defined as an atom or molecule with one or more unpaired electrons in its outer orbitals that is capable of independent existence.) The superoxide radical is not a powerful oxidant (hence the "superoxide" moniker seems undeserved), but it can be cytotoxic by virtue of its secondary actions (e.g., the reaction with nitric oxide described below). There is evidence that the superoxide radical is a major source of inflammatory pain (2), which infers that it is also a source of inflammatory tissue injury.

Reaction with Nitric Oxide

The superoxide radical readily reacts with nitric oxide (NO˙), a celebrated free radical (and the Molecule of the Year in 1992!) that promotes circulatory blood flow via vasodilation and inhibition of platelet aggregation (3). The reaction of these two radicals produces a nonradical, peroxynitrite ($ONOO^-$):

$$NO^{\cdot} + O_2^{\cdot} \rightarrow ONOO^- \qquad (8.3)$$

This reaction has two adverse consequences:

1. It attenuates the salutary effects of nitric oxide and promotes vasoconstriction and reduced blood flow. This vasoconstrictor effect has been used to explain the association between atherosclerosis (where the underlying inflammation produces superoxide in abundance) and hypertension (4). It is also the proposed mechanism for the vasoconstrictor effects of O_2 (see Chapter 4).
2. It produces peroxynitrite, a potent oxidizing agent capable of oxidative cell injury (3,4).

Hydrogen Peroxide

The addition of a single electron to the superoxide radical converts it to a peroxide ion, which has no unpaired electrons (see Figure 8.2). The addition of two protons (H^+) then produces hydrogen peroxide (H_2O_2); i.e.:

$$O_2^{\cdot} + e^- + 2\,H^+ \rightarrow H_2O_2 \qquad (8.4)$$

The electron donor for this reaction is another superoxide radical, so the overall reaction is:

$$2\,O_2^{\cdot} + 2\,H+ \rightarrow H_2O_2 + O_2 \qquad (8.5)$$

This is a *dismutation* reaction, which is a reaction in which the same chemical species is both oxidized and reduced. (In this case, superoxide radicals both donate and accept electrons.) This reaction is almost instantaneous when catalyzed by the enzyme *superoxide dismutase*. (This enzyme is an endogenous antioxidant, and is described in Chapter 12.)

Hydrogen peroxide is not a free radical (i.e., it has no unpaired electrons), and it is not a powerful oxidizing agent. However, it is very mobile and readily crosses cell membranes, where it can generate toxic hydroxyl radicals (see next). This explains why H_2O_2 can produce DNA strand breaks when added to cell cultures, but not when added to isolated DNA preparations (4,5).

Hydroxyl Radical

The single-electron reduction of H_2O_2 produces a powerful oxidant known as the hydroxyl radical, and the electron donor is iron

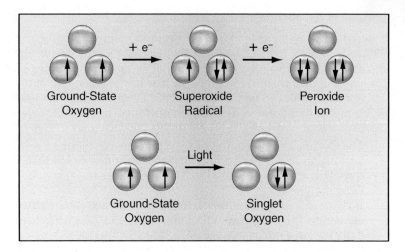

FIGURE 8.2 Electron configuration in the outer orbitals of ground-state oxygen and its derivatives. Circles denote atomic orbitals, and arrows represent electrons and their directional spin. See text for further explanation.

in a reduced state (Fe^{2+}). The reaction is as follows:

$$H_2O_2 + Fe^{2+} \rightarrow Fe^{3+} + OH^{\cdot} + OH^{-} \qquad (8.6)$$

where Fe^{2+} is ferrous (reduced) iron, Fe^{3+} is ferric (oxidized) iron, $OH^{\cdot}$ is the hydroxyl radical, and OH^{-} is the hydroxyl ion. This reaction is known as the *Fenton reaction*, and the oxidation of organic substrates by this reaction is known as *Fenton chemistry* (6). (The importance of iron as a source of oxidative cell injury is described later in the chapter.)

The hydroxyl radical is one the most reactive chemical species known, and often reacts with the first molecule it encounters (4). This highly reactive nature limits the mobility of hydroxyl radicals, but their range of destruction is expanded by H_2O_2, which can travel widely throughout the body and generate hydroxyl radicals wherever ferrous (Fe^{2+}) iron is available. This scenario has been implicated in the widespread reperfusion injury that can follow cardiopulmonary resuscitation (7).

The final reaction in O_2 metabolism is the single-electron reduction of the hydroxyl radical, which produces water:

$$OH^{\cdot} + OH^{-} + e^{-} + 2\,H^{+} \rightarrow 2\,H_2O \qquad (8.7)$$

Leakage of Metabolites

The reduction of O_2 to H_2O in mitochondria is complete in about 98% of instances. In the remaining 2% of cases, O_2 is incompletely metabolized to a reactive metabolite that escapes the confines of cytochrome oxidase and can do harm. The low leakage rate of reactive metabolites can be misleading because of the large volume of O_2 metabolized daily. This is demonstrated in the following calculations:

1. The O_2 consumption (VO_2) of an adult at rest is about 3.5 mL/kg/min, and for a 70 kg adult, this is 245 mL/min, or 353 liters/day. This corresponds to 353/22.4 = 15.7 moles of O_2 metabolized daily.
2. If 2% of 15.7 moles (0.3 moles) forms reactive metabolites that escape the mitochondria, this amounts to 0.3 x 32 = 9.6 grams daily (using a molar mass of 32 for the O_2 molecule).
3. Over a one-year period, the leakage of reactive metabolites would be 365 x 9.6 = 3.5 kg, which is 5% of the body weight (70 kg).

Thus, the cumulative leakage of reactive metabolites is far greater than suspected from the 2% leakage rate.

OTHER SOURCES

Oxygen metabolism in mitochondria is not the sole source of reactive oxygen species (ROS), nor is it the principal source of ROS in specific conditions (e.g., inflammation). The following is a brief description of other notable sources of ROS.

NADPH Oxidase

The major source of nonmitochondrial ROS production is an oxidase enzyme on the outer surface of cell membranes that promotes the addition of a single electron to O_2 to produce superoxide radicals. The electron donor for this reaction is NADPH; hence, the enzyme is called *NADPH oxidase*, commonly abbreviated as *NOX*. The NOX reaction is shown below:

$$O_2 + NADPH \rightarrow O_2^\cdot + NADP + H^+ \qquad (8.8)$$

This oxidase reaction is similar to the cytochrome oxidase reaction that initiates O_2 metabolism in mitochondria (see Equation 8.2), the only difference being the electron donor. NOX-generated superoxide radicals are extracellular in location and can be reduced further to form hydrogen peroxide and hypochlorous acid, a powerful microbicidal agent (see Chapter 9).

Table 8.2   The Variety of NADPH Oxidases

Location	Trigger	Consequences
Neutrophils, Macrophages	Cytokines	• Neutrophil activation • Phagocytosis • Tissue injury
Endothelium	Cytokines	• Increased vascular permeability • Increased leukocyte adhesion • Increased platelet adhesion • Microvascular thrombosis
	Oxidized LDL	• Atherosclerosis
Vascular Smooth Muscle	Angiotensin II	• Vasoconstriction • Hypertension
Airway Epithelium	Cytokines Allergens	• Airway hyperreactivity

Multiple Roles

Membrane-bound NOX enzymes are found in a wide variety of cells, including phagocytes, endothelial cells, vascular smooth muscle, adipocytes, and epithelial cells in the airways and large bowel (9). These enzymes are normally inactive, and both the triggering stimulus and functional role of the enzyme can vary in each type of cell. Some examples of this variety are shown in Table 8.2. The most studied role of NOX enzymes is in the acute inflammatory response, where they are responsible for neutrophil activation and increased vascular permeability (9,10). (The role of NOX enzymes in the inflammatory response is described in detail in Chapter 9.) NOX enzymes also participate in a variety of physiological control responses, where the production of ROS serves as a "signal" of an abnormal condition that requires correction. The participation of ROS in physiological control responses is described later in the chapter.

Xanthine Oxidase

The final steps in the degradation of purine nucleotides (adenine and guanine) is the conversion of hypoxanthine to xanthine, and xanthine to uric acid (see Figure 8.3). These reactions are oxidations (i.e., involve loss of electrons), and the fate of the released electrons is determined by the redox state of the tissues. When conditions are normal, the oxidations are catalyzed by the enzyme xanthine dehydrogenase (XDH), and the released electrons are transferred to its cofactor, nicotinamide adenine nucleotide (NAD). However, in conditions where the redox balance favors oxidation (e.g., inflammation), XDH is converted to xanthine oxidase (XO), and this enzyme transfers the electrons to the O_2 molecule to generate superoxide radicals, which are readily converted to hydrogen peroxide. Thus, the predominant end product of XO-catalyzed purine degradation is hydrogen peroxide (12).

Ischemia-Reperfusion Injury

Animal studies have shown that allopurinol (an XO inhibitor) reduces the severity of ischemia-reperfusion injury (13), and this observation has fueled the following proposed scenario. During periods of ischemia, ATP stores are depleted, and AMP is degraded to hypoxanthine. When flow is reestablished, the reperfused areas become inflamed, and this promotes the conversion of XDH to XO. The actions of XO on the accumulated hypoxanthine creates a surge in the production of hydrogen peroxide, which then damages the endothelium (via the production of hydroxyl radicals).

Singlet Oxygen

The O_2 molecule can be raised to a higher energy state by the input of energy, which causes one of the unpaired electrons to flip its directional spin and form an appropriate match with the other unpaired electron. The resulting electron configuration, which is shown in Figure 8.2, is known as *singlet oxygen* (4).

Photosensitivity

Light is the major source of energy for singlet O_2 production. The light first reacts with photosensitizer molecules that absorb specific wavelengths of light, and the energized photosensitizer then transfers the energy to ground-state O_2 to produce singlet O_2. There are a variety of sensitizers, including riboflavin (B6), flavine nucleotides (FAD, FMN), pigments (bilirubin, and porphyrins), dyes (e.g., methylene blue, toluidine blue), and drugs (e.g., phenothiazines, fluoroquinolones) (4).

Singlet O_2 is a powerful oxidant that can damage membrane lipids, nucleic acids, and proteins, and the principal organs involved

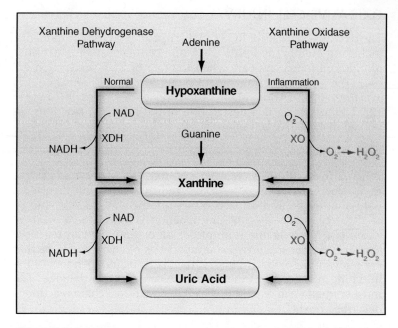

FIGURE 8.3 The terminal reactions in the metabolism of purine nucleotides (adenine and guanine). The normal catalyst for these reactions is xanthine dehydrogenase (XDH), but in the setting of inflammation, the catalyst is xanthine oxidase (XO), which produces superoxide radicals ($O_2^{\cdot}$) and hydrogen peroxide (H_2O_2).

are the skin and eyes. Photosensitive skin lesions can vary from mild erythema to bullae, scarring, and disfigurement. Skin lesions are a prominent feature of the porphyrias (14) because of the photosensitizing actions of the porphyrins and their tendency to accumulate in the skin. The eye is susceptible to photic injury because of the light-sensitive pigment, rhodopsin, located in the rods. A familiar example of oxidant-mediated retinal injury is *retinitis pigmentosa,* which causes premature damage in the rods of the retina (where rhodopsin is located).

Quenching

Singlet O_2 can transfer its energy to another molecule and convert back to ground-state O_2. This is known as *quenching,* and the molecule that receives the energy is called a *scavenger.* An effective scavenger for singlet O_2 is β-carotene (4).

OXIDATIVE CELL INJURY

The oxidative actions of ROS can disrupt all vital cell components, including membrane lipids DNA and cellular proteins. This oxidative cell injury appears when the rate of ROS production exceeds the capacity for antioxidant protection; a condition known as *oxidative stress*. (Antioxidant protection is described in Chapter 12.) The following is a description of the principal reactions involved in oxidative cell injury.

Chain Reactions

When a free radical reacts with a nonradical, the nonradical loses an electron and becomes a free radical, which can then react with another nonradical to produce another free radical, and so on. This type of self-sustaining reaction is known as a *chain reaction* (4). A fire is one example of an oxidative chain reaction, and fires demonstrate two characteristics of chain reactions that are relevant for oxidative injury: they become independent of the initiating reaction, and they produce considerable damage. The most studied form of oxidative cell injury from a chain reaction is described next.

Lipid Peroxidation

The hydrophobic interior of cell membranes is populated by polyunsaturated fatty acids (PUFAs), which promote the "fluidity" of cell membranes by virtue of their low melting point (15). (PUFAs are also used to promote fluidity in cooking oils and paints.) PUFAs are particularly susceptible to oxidative disruption; a process known as *lipid peroxidation*, which produces *rancidity* when it involves PUFAs in food products (as described in Chapter 7). When lipid peroxidation occurs in cell membranes, the PUFAs polymerize and lose their fluidity, causing membranes to become stiff and lose their selective permeability. This results in leaky cell membranes, which culminates in the osmotic disruption of cells.

The Reaction Sequence

Lipid peroxidation is especially destructive because it proceeds as a self-sustaining chain reaction. The reaction sequence is shown in Figure 8.4. The initial event is a strong oxidant like the hydroxyl radical that removes an entire hydrogen atom from one of the carbon atoms of a PUFA. This creates a carbon-centered lipid radical, which reacts with O_2 to form an oxygen-centered "peroxyl radical." Propagation occurs when the peroxyl radical removes a hydrogen atom from an adjacent PUFA, which initiates a new series of reactions, while also producing a lipid hydroperoxide. This repetition will continue until the substrate (PUFA) is exhausted, or something blocks the propagation. (Vitamin E blocks the propagation of lipid peroxidation, as described in Chapter 12.)

An additional method of propagation occurs when ferrous iron (Fe^{2+}) is available and reacts with the lipid hydroperoxide (LOOH) produced by the propagation reaction. This reaction splits the oxygen-oxygen bond in LOOH and produces another free radical, the *alkoxyl radical* (LO˙), as shown below.

$$LOOH + Fe^{2+} \rightarrow Fe^{3+} + LO˙ + OH^- \qquad (8.9)$$

(Note the similarity between this reaction and the Fenton reaction in equation 8.6.) Alkoxyl radicals can remove a hydrogen atom from PUFAs and initiate lipid peroxidation. Iron-initiated lipid peroxidation has been identified as a type of regulated cell death known as *ferroptosis* (17).

DNA Damage

The constant threat of oxidative damage from ROS is demonstrated in studies that show the presence of oxidative DNA damage during normal metabolism (15,18). *The rate of oxidative damage in*

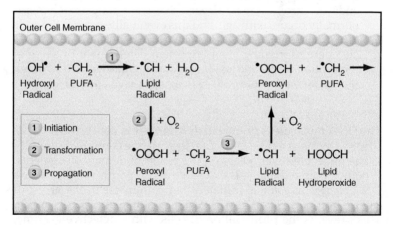

FIGURE 8.4 The reaction sequence for lipid peroxidation in cell membranes, which propagates as a self-sustaining "chain reaction." Free radicals are indicated by a superscripted dot. PUFA = polyunsaturated fatty acid. See text for explanation.

DNA has been estimated at 500,000 – 2 million molecular "lesions" per cell per day (18), with rates in the higher range of normal expected in highly oxidative organs (e.g., brain). Hydroxyl radicals are the principal source of oxidative DNA damage (15). Hydrogen peroxide can be a source of widespread DNA damage, but only by virtue of producing hydroxyl radicals wherever it travels (see Equation 8.6).

There are three forms of oxidative DNA damage (19), which are summarized below (see Figure 8.5).

1. Oxidation modifies nucleotide bases (adenine, guanine, cytosine, and thymine), which can alter gene expression. Guanine is particularly susceptible to oxidative modification, and detection of oxidized guanine residues (8-oxo-2-deoxyguanosine) is a popular method of monitoring oxidative damage in DNA (18).

2. The covalent bonds that link nucleotides together are disrupted by oxidation. These are called "DNA strand breaks," and they can involve one or both polynucleotide chains. Single strand breaks can often be repaired, but disruptions in both polynucleotide chains (double strand breaks) are difficult to repair.

3. Oxidation promotes the shortening of *telomeres*, which are repetitive sequences of nucleotide bases that wrap around the ends of chromosomes. Progressive shortening of telomeres normally occurs with age, and this eventually exposes the ends of chromosomes, which prevents further cell replication (20). Telomere shortening is an important determinant of aging at the cellular level, and oxidative damage hastens this process. (For more on the role of ROS in aging, see Chapter 11.)

Consequences

The DNA molecule is unique in that damage is not corrected by *de novo* synthesis of a new molecule. Instead, the continued integrity of the molecule relies solely on the repair of damaged segments. When oxidative damage is extensive and repair is not possible, a *DNA damage response* is initiated that culminates in the arrest of cell replication (*replicative senescence*) or cell death (*apoptosis*) (19). This prevents the proliferation of cells with a defective genome, but hastens the process of aging. (The DNA damage response is described in more detail in Chapter 11.) On the other hand, damage involving select genes (e.g., tumor suppressor gene) can lead to uncontrolled proliferation and neoplastic transformation.

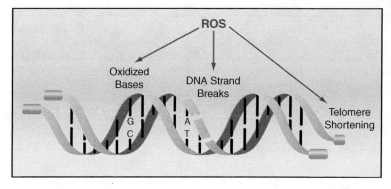

FIGURE 8.5 Three types of oxidative damage to the DNA molecule. ROS = reactive oxygen species. A, C, G, T = adenine, cytosine, guanine, thymine, respectively. See text for explanation.

Protein Degradation

Oxidative damage can alter protein function in three ways:

1. Oxidation disrupts the covalent bonds that hold polypeptides together. This process is usually initiated by hydroxyl radicals, and it proceeds as a chain reaction, with the same type of reaction sequence described for lipid peroxidation (21). Disrupted polypeptides then become more susceptible to the actions of proteases.
2. Oxidation can alter the behavior of all 20 amino acids, with aromatic amino acids (phenylalanine, tryptophan, tyrosine, and histidine) being most susceptible (18).
3. Protein modification can be a secondary phenomenon; i.e., when oxidative DNA damage results in the production of faulty proteins.

The consequences of protein modification are as legion as the multitude of proteins and their associated functions. For example, there are an estimated 75,000 different enzymes in the human body (22), and any or all of these enzymes can be modified by oxidation.

IRON

Iron has a perplexing relationship with O_2 because it transports O_2 to tissues (as the iron in hemoglobin), yet it plays a major role in O_2-related cell injury. Table 8.3 includes some of the diseases in which iron-related cell injury has been implicated.

TABLE 8.3	Diseases in Which Iron-related Injury Plays a Role
Organ	**Disease**
Central Nervous System (CNS)	• Ischemic Stroke • Traumatic Brain Injury • Huntington Disease
Heart	• Cardiomyopathy from ischemia-reperfusion, and chemotherapy
Vascular System	• Atherosclerosis • Endothelial injury from ischemia-reperfusion • Endothelial injury and vascular occlusion in DIC and sickle cell disease
Kidneys	• Acute kidney injury from myoglobinuria and ischemia-reperfusion • Chromophobe renal cell carcinoma
Pancreas	• Gestational diabetes
Liver	• Hemochromatosis

Properties

Iron is highly oxidizable and has a total of 5 oxidation states: Fe^{2+} to Fe^{6+} (23). The most common ones are Fe^{2+} (ferrous iron) and Fe^{3+} (ferric iron), which are formed from ground-state iron (Fe) by the sequential removal of electrons (e^-):

$$Fe - 2e^- \rightarrow Fe^{2+} - e^- \rightarrow Fe^{3+} \qquad (8.10)$$

Ferrous iron (Fe^{2+}) is present in hemoglobin and myoglobin (where it binds O_2) and is the single-electron donor in the production of hydroxyl radicals from H_2O_2 (Equation 8.6). Ferric iron (Fe^{3+}) is the storage form of iron (and is bound to ferritin and hemosiderin) and is also present in methemoglobin and metmyoglobin (where it does not bind O_2).

Another property of iron that deserves mention is the presence of unpaired electrons: Fe^{2+} has 4 unpaired electrons, and there are 5 unpaired electrons in Fe^{3+} (8). This allows both forms of iron to trigger chain reactions when they react with a nonradical.

Iron and Oxidative Cell Injury

Iron plays a major role in oxidative cell injury because of its participation in the production of hydroxyl radicals (see Equation 8.6), the most damaging of the ROS (24). Iron is also capable of directly initiating the oxidation of membrane lipids (see Equation 8.9).

Ferroptosis

As mentioned earlier, iron-induced lipid peroxidation can serve as a form of regulated cell death known as ferroptosis (17). This form of lipid peroxidation is triggered by inflammation, and it has been implicated in the pathogenesis of ischemic kidney injury, ischemic and chemotherapy-induced cardiomyopathy, and ischemic stroke (25-27).

Heme Iron

Heme-derived iron plays an important role in endothelial damage from hemolysis (e.g., sickle cell disease and DIC) and in ischemia-reperfusion injury (28). The heme released from red blood cells is hydrophobic, and inserts itself in endothelial cell membranes, where the release of ferrous iron (Fe^{2+}) can trigger lipid peroxidation. The same process has been implicated in the damage of renal tubular cells by myoglobinuria (28), and in the brain injury associated with intracranial hemorrhage (29).

Iron Sequestration

The importance of iron as a source of oxidative cell injury is suggested by the extensive protein binding of iron. There is an abundance of iron in the human body (50 mg/kg for an adult male, and 20-25% less for a premenopausal woman), and almost all of it is bound to proteins: about 65% is bound to hemoglobin, 10% is bound to myoglobin and iron-dependent enzymes (e.g., cytochrome P-450 family of enzymes), 20-30% is bound to ferritin and hemosiderin in tissues, and the small amount of iron in plasma (65-165 µg/dL) is bound to transferrin (30). This leaves *little or no free (unbound) iron,* which protects against iron-induced cell injury.

Anemia of Inflammation

Another type of protective iron sequestration is the anemia that develops in response to systemic inflammation. The iron needed for erythropoiesis is provided by macrophages, and iron release by macrophages is inhibited in the setting of systemic inflammation (by an iron-regulating hormone known as *hepsidin*) (30). The decrease in available iron eventually leads to the *anemia of inflammation* (formerly known as the "anemia of chronic disease") (31). The *anemia of critical illness* (32) is the acute form of this disorder. This type of anemia is associated with a decrease in serum iron, which is advantageous in an oxidation-prone condition like inflammation.

PHYSIOLOGICAL ROLE

The role of ROS as a source of pathological injury occurs primarily during periods of oxidative stress, when there is an abundance of ROS, or a deficiency in antioxidant protection, or both. However as mentioned earlier, ROS can also participate in physiological control responses during "normal" metabolism . This condition in which low doses of a toxic substance provide a benefit is known as *hormesis* (33). Some examples of this are presented here. Note that the ROS in these cases originate from the membrane-bound NADPH oxidase (NOX) enzyme, and are not mitochondrial in origin.

Oxygen Sensing

The red blood cell mass is maintained by the hormone erythropoietin, which is produced in the kidney and liver in response to hypoxemia. Hydrogen peroxide inhibits this response by degrading a transcriptional protein (hypoxia-inducible-factor-1) that stimulates erythropoietin production (11). These observations have led to the theory that the oxygen tension in blood is sensed by the production of ROS from endothelial cells in the liver and kidneys (via the NOX enzyme on the endothelial cell membrane), and that a decrease in ROS production by these cells is responsible for the erythropoietin response to hypoxemia. This mechanism has also been implicated in the response to hypoxemia by chemoreceptors in the carotid body (11).

Glycemic Control

Insulin induces the production of H_2O_2 by activation of an NOX enzyme in the cell membrane of adipocytes (34), and physiological concentrations of H_2O_2 have been shown to enhance insulin responsiveness (35). These two observations indicate that, under normal conditions, H_2O_2 has a permissive role in the maintenance of euglycemia by insulin. This contrasts with the role of H_2O_2 during periods of oxidative stress, where it promotes the development of complications associated with diabetes (e.g., atherosclerosis).

Vascular Control

ROS have been implicated in vascular control by the renin-angio-tensin-aldosterone system (36). During low-flow states, angiotensin-induced vasoconstriction helps to maintain blood pressure. This vasoconstrictor effect may be mediated by ROS, because angiotensin activates the NOX enzyme in vascular smooth muscle, and the subsequent production of superoxide radicals can produce vasoconstriction by inactivating nitric oxide (see Equation 8.3).

SUMMATION

The major points in this chapter are summarized as follows:

1. The destructive actions of oxygen *in vivo* are carried out by a group of reactive chemical derivatives, known as reactive oxygen species (ROS). These include the superoxide radical, hydrogen peroxide, the hydroxyl radical, and singlet oxygen.
2. There are three major types of oxidative cell injury:
   a. Oxidation of membrane lipids alters the viscoelastic properties of membranes, which leads to loss of selective membrane permeability and eventual osmotic disruption of cells.
   b. Oxidative damage of DNA can include strand breaks, modification of nucleotide bases, and accelerated shortening of telomeres. The consequences of these reactions include genomic aberrations (including neoplastic transformations), cessation of cell replication, and premature cell death.
   c. Oxidation promotes protein degradation, which can have a wide variety of adverse consequences (depending on the protein involved).
3. Iron plays an important role in oxidative cell injury because it promotes the formation of highly destructive hydroxyl radicals. The destructive potential of iron explains why almost all the iron in the body is bound and sequestered.
4. Oxidative cell injury occurs predominantly during periods of oxidative stress, when the production of ROS exceeds the capacity for antioxidant protection. During periods of "normal metabolism" (with no oxidative stress), ROS may participate in physiological control responses.

REFERENCES

a. Walford RL. Maximum Life Span. New York: W.W. Norton and Co, 1983:87.

1. Grisham MB. Reactive oxygen metabolism. In: Reactive Metabolites of Oxygen and Nitrogen in Biology and Medicine. Austin, TX: R.G. Landes Co., 1991:5-19.
2. Wand Z-Q, Porreca F, Cuzzocrea S, et al. A newly identified role for superoxide in inflammatory pain. J Pharmacol Exp Therap 2004; 309:869-878.
3. Radi R. Oxygen radicals, nitric oxide, and peroxynitrite: Redox pathways in molecular medicine. Proc Nat Acad Sci 2018; 115:5839-5848.
4. Halliwell B, Gutteridge JMC. Redox chemistry: the essentials. In: Free Radicals in Biology and Medicine. 5th ed, Oxford: Oxford University Press, 2015:30-76.
5. Spragg RG. DNA strand break formation following exposure of bovine pulmonary artery and aortic endothelial cells to reactive oxygen products. Am J Respir Cell Mol Biol 1991; 4:4-10.
6. Barbusinski, K. Fenton reaction – controversies concerning the chemistry. Ecol Chem Engin 2009; 16:347-358.
7. Huet O, Dupic L, Batteux F, et al. Postresuscitation syndrome: potential role of hydroxyl radical-induced endothelial cell damage. Crit Care Med 2011; 39:1712-1720.
8. Halliwell B, Gutteridge JMC. Free Radicals in Biology and Medicine. 5th ed, Oxford: Oxford University Press, 2015:1-29.
9. Bedard K, Krause KH. The NOX family of ROS-generating NADPH oxidases: physiology and pathophysiology. Physiol Rev 2007; 87:245-313.
10. Mittal M, Siddiqui MR, Tran K, et al. Reactive oxygen species in inflammation and tissue injury. Antiox Redox Sig 2014; 20:1126-1167.
11. Dröge W. Free radicals in the physiological control of cell function. Physiol Rev 2002; 82:47-95.
12. Kelley EE, Khoo NKH, Hundley NJ, et al. Hydrogen peroxide is the major oxidant product of xanthine oxidase. Free Radic Biol Med 2010; 48:493-498.
13. Halliwell B, Gutteridge JMC. Reactive species in disease: friends or foes? In: Free Radicals in Biology and Medicine. 5th ed, Oxford: Oxford University Press, 2015:511-638.
14. Puy H, Gouya L, Deybach JC. Porphyrias. Lancet 2010; 375:924937.
15. Halliwell B, Gutteridge JMC. Oxidative stress and redox regulation: adaptation, damage, repair, senescence, and death. In: Free Radicals in Biology and Medicine. 5th ed, Oxford: Oxford University Press, 2015:199-283.
16. Shahidi F, Zhong Y. Lipid oxidation and improving the oxidative stability. Chem Soc Rev 2010; 39:4067-4079.

17. Yang WS, Stockwell BR. Ferroptosis: death by lipid peroxidation. Trends Cell Biol 2016; 26:165-176.
18. Hamilton ML, Van Remmen H, Drake JA, et al. Does oxidative damage to DNA increase with age? Proc Natl Acad Sci 2001; 98:10469-10474.
19. Jan HJ, Hoeijmakers. DNA damage, aging, and cancer. New Engl J Med 2009; 361:1475-1485.
20. Shay JW. Telomeres and aging. Curr Opin Cell Biol 2018; 52:1-7.
21. Stadtman ER. Protein modification. In: Banerjee R, ed. Redox Biochemistry. New York, John Wiley & Sons, 2008:184-194.
22. Svarney T, Barnes-Svarney P. The Handy Biology Answer Book. 2nd ed. Canton, MI: Visible Ink Press, 2014.
23. Zhuang T, Han H, Yang Z. Iron, oxidative stress, and gestational diabetes. Nutrients 2014; 6:3968-3980.
24. Menegheni R. Iron homeostasis, oxidative stress, and DNA damage. Free Rad Biol Med 1997; 23:783-792.
25. Feng X, Wang H, Han D, et al. Ferroptosis as a target for protection against cardiomyopathy. Proc Nat Acad Sci 2019; 116:2672-2680.
26. Muller T, Dewitz C, Schmitz J, et al. Necroptosis and ferroptosis are alternative cell death pathways that operate in acute kidney failure. Cell Mol Life Sci 2017; 74:3631-3645.
27. Linkermann A, Stockwell BR, Krautwald S, Anders HJ. Regulated cell death and inflammation: an auto-amplification loop causes organ failure. Nat Rev Immunol 2014; 14:759-767.
28. Belcher JD, Beckman JD, Balla G, et al. Heme degradation and vascular injury. Antiox Redox Signal 2010; 12:233-248.
29. Garton T, Keep RF, Hua Y, Xi G. Brain iron overload following intracranial hemorrhage. Stroke Vasc Neurol 2016; 1:e000042.
30. Gisbert JP, Gomollon F. An update on iron physiology. World J Gastroenterol 2009; 15:4617-4626.
31. Ganz T, Nemeth E. Iron sequestration and anemia of inflammation. Semin Hematol 2009; 46:387-393.
32. Corwin HL, Krantz SB. Anemia of the critically ill: "acute" anemia of chronic disease. Crit Care Med 2000; 28:3098-3099.
33. Mattson MP. Hormesis defined. Ageing Res Rev 2008; 7:1-7.
34. Kreiger-Brauer H, Medda PK, Kather H. Insulin-induced activation of NADPH-dependent H_2O_2 generation in human adipocyte plasma membranes is mediated by $G\alpha12$. J Biol Chem 1997; 272:10135-10142.
35. Schmid E, Hotz-Wagenblatt A, Dröge W. Phosphorylation of the insulin receptor kinase by phosphocreatine in combination with hydrogen peroxide. The structural basis of redox priming. FASEB J; 1999:13:1491-1500.
36. Schramm A, Matusik P, Osmenda G, Guzik TJ. Targeting NADPH oxidases in vascular pharmacology. Vasc Pharmacol 2012; 56:216-231.

Does oxygen participate in the inflammatory response?

9

"Inflammation itself is not considered a disease but a salutary operation…
but when it cannot accomplish that salutary purpose…it does mischief."

John Hunter, MD

The author of the introductory quote was a preeminent 18th-century Scottish surgeon whose observations on inflammation became the accepted wisdom on the subject for most of the 19th century (1). His comment on the ability of inflammation to do harm was prescient, as inflammation is now recognized as a major factor in a multitude of pathological conditions, like those listed in Table 9.1. Considering the scope of these disease entities, inflammation deserves recognition as a leading source of morbidity and mortality in modern times. Also deserving of this recognition is oxygen and its more reactive offspring (i.e., the reactive oxygen species introduced in the last chapter), because they play a major role in the inflammatory response (2), as described in this chapter.

NEUTROPHIL ACTIVATION

In the initial stages of the inflammatory response, neutrophils (and other granulocytes) experience a precipitous rise in O_2 consumption (up to 20-fold) that lasts for 15-20 minutes (3). This is known as the *respiratory burst*, which is a misnomer, because the surge in O_2 consumption does not take place in mitochondria, and does not produce high-energy ATP molecules. Instead, the respiratory burst generates reactive oxygen species (ROS), which are used to kill invading microbes. The trigger for this reaction is activation of an NADPH oxidase (NOX) enzyme located on the outer surface of the neutrophil cell membrane. (NOX enzymes are introduced in Chapter 8, and their multiple functions are shown in Table 8.2.) This enzyme catalyzes the single-electron reduction of O_2 to form the superoxide radical ($O_2^{\cdot}$), with NADPH as the electron donor:

$$O_2 + NADPH \rightarrow O_2^{\cdot} + NADP + H^+ \qquad (9.1)$$

123

TABLE 9.1   Diseases in Which Inflammation Plays a Major Role

Acute	Chronic
ACS	Alzheimer Disease
ARDS	Atherosclerosis
Anaphylaxis	Autoimmune Diseases
Asthma	Cardiomyopathy (ischemic)
COP	COPD
Hepatitis (noninfectious)	Diabetes (type II)
Interstitial nephritis	Inflammatory Bowel Disease
Pancreatitis	Interstitial Lung Disease
Radiation Pneumonitis	Macular Degeneration
Reperfusion Injury	Neurodegenerative Disorders
Sepsis with Multiorgan Failure	Occupational Lung Disease
TRALI	Osteoarthritis
TTP	Parkinson Disease

Abbreviations: ACS = acute coronary syndrome, ARDS = acute respiratory distress syndrome, COP = cryptogenic organizing pneumonia, TRALI = transfusion-related acute lung injury, TTP = thrombotic thrombocytopenia purpura, COPD = chronic obstructive pulmonary disease.

These superoxide radicals are generated extracellularly (see Figure 9.1), to combat invading microbes. This action is not attributed to the superoxide radicals themselves, but to the propensity of superoxide radicals to combine and form hydrogen peroxide (H_2O_2); i.e.,

$$2O_2^{\cdot} + 2H^+ \rightarrow H_2O_2 + O_2 \qquad (9.2)$$

As mentioned in Chapter 8, this is a *dismutation reaction,* which is a reaction in which the same chemical species is both oxidized and reduced. (In this case, superoxide radicals both donate and accept electrons.) This reaction is almost instantaneous when catalyzed by the enzyme superoxide dismutase. Hydrogen peroxide is both microbicidal and cytotoxic, but these effects are primarily due to the production of more toxic chemical species (see next).

Hypochlorous Acid

The cytoplasmic granules in neutrophils are rich in the enzyme myeloperoxidase, which is released by the degranulation of neutrophils. This enzyme promotes the chlorination of hydrogen peroxide (H_2O_2) to form hypochlorous acid (HOCL):

$$H_2O_2 + CL^- + H^+ \rightarrow HOCL + H_2O \qquad (9.3)$$

This reaction accounts for about 30% of the O_2 consumed during the respiratory burst (3).

The end product, HOCL, is a potent oxidizing agent that has bactericidal, fungicidal, and viricidal activity. (Sodium hypochlorite, the sodium salt of HOCL, is the principal ingredient in household bleach.) In addition to its microbicidal effects, HOCL plays a major role in inflammatory tissue injury (see later).

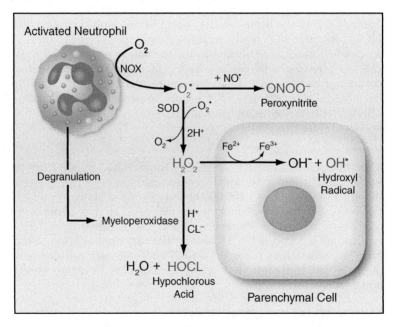

FIGURE 9.1 The chemical reactions triggered by activation of the NADPH oxidase enzyme (NOX) in the cell membrane of neutrophils. SOD = superoxide dismutase. See text for explanation.

Hydroxyl Radical

Hydrogen peroxide can also accept a single electron from iron (Fe^{2+}) to form the highly destructive hydroxyl radical; i.e.,

$$H_2O_2 + Fe^{2+} \rightarrow Fe^{3+} + OH^{\cdot} + OH^{-} \qquad (9.4)$$

Fe^{2+} is ferrous (reduced) iron, Fe^{3+} is ferric (oxidized) iron, $OH^{\cdot}$ is the hydroxyl radical, and OH^{-} is the hydroxyl ion. This reaction is not favored in the extracellular fluid because of the paucity of free iron. However, hydrogen peroxide can readily enter cells and generate hydroxyl radicals whenever it encounters ferrous iron. This is a prominent source of oxidative cell injury and is also an important mechanism for microbial killing by phagocytosis.

Phagocytosis

Phagocytosis is considered the first line of defense against invading microbes. The location of the NOX enzyme in the outer portion of the cell membrane is well-suited for phagocytosis; i.e., when the cell membrane invaginates to engulf microbes, the enzyme is facing the lumen of the "phagosome,"and this gives the NOX-generated ROS ready access to the microbes (see Figure 9.2). Microbial killing is attributed to the formation of hydroxyl radicals from hydrogen peroxide, which is facilitated by the high iron content of bacteria (4). This is the same mechanism of action for bactericidal antibiotics (5). HOCL can also participate in microbial killing in phagosomes, but it is more involved in eradicating microbes in the extracellular space.

Chronic Granulomatous Disease

The antimicrobial impact of ROS is demonstrated by a condition known as chronic granulomatous disease. This is a rare genetic disorder (incidence is 1:200,000 births in United States) in which the NOX enzyme in phagocytes is defective, and patients with this disorder suffer from recurrent and life-threatening bacterial and fungal infections (7). Moreover, the functional deficit of the NOX enzyme varies (from 0.1% to 27% of normal) in individual patients, and those with less severe deficits have fewer infections and survive longer (8).

ENDOTHELIAL DYSFUNCTION

The endothelium is more than a barrier between the bloodstream and parenchymal tissue, because it also has an active role in maintaining blood flow. The principal participant in this effort is nitric oxide, a free radical (classified as a "reactive nitrogen species")

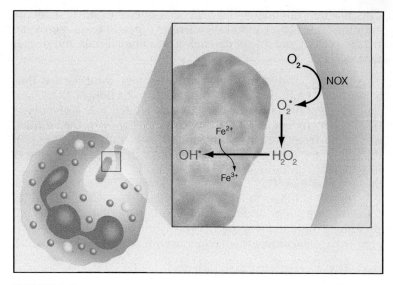

FIGURE 9.2 The principal mechanism of microbial killing by phagocytosis. See text for explanation.

produced in endothelial cells and vascular smooth muscle that promotes vasodilation and prevents the adhesion of leukocytes and platelets to the endothelial surface (9). The inflammatory response alters the behavior of the endothelium: i.e., leukocytes and platelets adhere to the endothelial surface, and the tight junctions between endothelial cells are disrupted, allowing leukocytes and other products of inflammation to move into affected tissues (2). These changes are adaptive, but they can also be deleterious, because the increase in platelet adhesiveness promotes microvascular thrombosis, and the disrupted endothelial barrier can result in excessive edema.

Role of ROS

The inciting event in the endothelial dysfunction associated with inflammation is activation of the NOX enzyme on the surface of endothelial cells (2,10). The subsequent production of superoxide radicals is instrumental in promoting leukocyte adhesion to the endothelium and in disrupting the tight junctions between endothelial cells. Part of this is a direct effect, and part is due to the reaction of superoxide radicals with nitric oxide ($NO^{\bullet}$):

$$O_2^{\bullet^-} + NO^{\bullet} \rightarrow ONOO^- \qquad (9.5)$$

This reaction eliminates the beneficial effects of nitric oxide on endothelial function and also generates a potent toxin, peroxynitrite ($ONOO^-$), capable of damaging endothelial cells and deeper tissues (11).

The endothelial dysfunction in inflammatory conditions is thus a result of "oxidative stress" (i.e., overproduction of ROS), and the degree of oxidative stress is directly related to the severity of disease. In studies using cultured endothelial cells, the addition of plasma from patients with septic shock stimulates ROS production in the cells, and the magnitude of the response is greater in patients with more severe disease and in patients who do not survive the illness (12). Continued ROS production by endothelial cells depletes intracellular antioxidants (13), and this magnifies the oxidative stress, and the risk of oxidative cell injury. This is a prelude to inflammatory multiorgan dysfunction, which is associated with lethal outcomes in patients with septic shock (see later).

INFLAMMATORY TISSUE INJURY

The concentration of ROS can reach as high as the millimolar range in areas of inflammation (9), and this creates a risk of oxidative damage in both the extracellular matrix and parenchymal cells. (*Note:* Not all of the ROS can be measured. Species like the superoxide radical and hydroxyl radical react almost instantaneously, so the products of their reactions are used to infer their presence.)

Extracellular Matrix

The extracellular matrix (ECM) is a complex mesh of proteins (e.g., collagen, elastin) and sugar-protein complexes (e.g., chondroitan sulfate) that differs in each of the major organs. The ECM is vulnerable to oxidative damage because the components have a slow turnover rate (14), and there is a paucity of antioxidant protection in extracellular fluids (15).

The major sources of oxidative damage in the ECM are peroxynitrite and myeloperoxidase (14). Peroxynitrite alters proteins in the ECM via "nitration," and this process has been implicated in several diseases, most notably Alzheimer disease (16) and Parkinson disease (17). Myeloperoxidase (MPO) binds to ECM proteins and creates a nidus for the production of HOCL, which readily oxidizes surrounding proteins (14). Oxidized proteins more readily bind MPO, which then leads to more protein oxidation, and this positive feedback system can result in widespread oxidative damage in the ECM (18). HOCL also inactivates α1-antiprotease (formerly α1-antitrypsin), which promotes the degradation of ECM proteins by protease enzymes (9). ECM damage from MPO and HOCL plays a major role in cardiovascular disease, as described in the last section of this chapter.

Inflammatory Pain

Animal studies of pain perception have shown that treatment with a superoxide dismutase mimetic (the enzyme that promotes the conversion of superoxide radicals to hydrogen peroxide) curtails the pain response to inflammation (19). This implicates superoxide radicals as a source of inflammatory pain; a finding supported by evidence that superoxide dismutase is inactivated by the inflammatory production of peroxynitrite (20), thereby promoting an overabundance of superoxide radicals in areas of inflammation. These findings have important implications for the development of nonopioid analgesics for painful inflammation.

Oxidative Cell Injury

Hydrogen peroxide can produce the highly destructive hydroxyl radicals in the ECM (see Figure 9.1), but this reaction is limited by the limited availability of free iron and by the decrease in extracellular iron that is associated with inflammation (21). However, a favored mechanism for oxidative cell injury is the movement of hydrogen peroxide into parenchymal cells, where it generates hydroxyl radicals whenever it encounters ferrous (Fe^{2+}) iron. Hydroxyl radicals are the most damaging of all the ROS, as described in Chapter 8.

Hypochlorous acid (HOCL) is also considered an important source of oxidative cell injury. HOCL oxidizes all types of organic molecules, but it especially targets the amino acid cysteine. Proteins that have cysteine in their active site are rapidly inactivated by HOCL, and these proteins include glutathione (the major intracellular antioxidant) and nitric oxide synthase (the source of nitric oxide) (22). Inactivation of both of these proteins will significantly magnify the risk of oxidative damage in inflammatory conditions.

INFLAMMATORY ROS AND DISEASE

The participation of ROS in the many facets of the inflammatory response is summarized in Table 9.2. It seems clear that ROS

TABLE 9.2   Participation of ROS in the Inflammatory Response

Component	ROS Involvement
Neutrophil activation	Respiratory burst is dedicated solely to ROS production
Leukocyte adherence to endothelium	Facilitated by NOX-generated ROS
Leukocyte movement across endothelium	Facilitated by NOX-generated ROS
Microbial killing	Hydroxyl radicals and hypochlorous acid are microbicidal
Extracellular matrix injury	Major factors are myeloperoxidase, hypochlorous acid and peroxynitrite
Inflammatory Pain	Superoxide radicals have a major role
Inflammatory Cell injury	Oxidative injury via hydroxyl radicals and hydrochlorous acid

NOX = NADPH oxidase enzyme.

are an essential feature of the inflammatory response, and have a major role in both the benefits (i.e., antimicrobial actions) and detrimental effects (i.e., tissue injury) of inflammation. This means that ROS also play a role in the multitude of inflammation-related diseases, such as those in Table 9.1. The following examples highlight the participation of "inflammatory ROS" in two of the most prevalent and lethal conditions in modern times.

Cardiovascular Disease

Cardiovascular disease is the dominant health concern in developed countries, and is perennially the leading cause of death in the United States (23). Inflammatory ROS are implicated in all forms of cardiovascular disease.

Atherosclerosis

The seminal condition in cardiovascular disease is atherosclerosis, a chronic inflammatory condition driven by the infiltration of neutrophils and macrophages into the subendothelial space of blood vessels (24). The process involves low-density lipoproteins

(LDLs), a transport vehicle for cholesterol that is 50% cholesterol, 25% protein (called apolipoprotein B) and 25% phospholipid. There is a well-documented association between levels of circulating LDL and the risk of coronary artery disease (25), but native LDL is not the problem. LDL accumulates in the subendothelial space, where it is oxidized by HOCL from activated neutrophils (26). The oxidized form of LDL is cytotoxic and is taken up by macrophages, creating the "foam cells" that are the hallmark of developing atheromas (27). Oxidized or "atherogenic" LDL also promotes leukocyte chemotaxis, which further perpetuates the localized inflammation. The participation of ROS in atherogenesis has been confirmed by studies showing that myeloperoxidase (MPO) is catalytically active in human atheromas, and that MPO is more abundant in advanced atheromatous plaques (22).

The atherosclerosis story also involves high-density lipoprotein (HDL), a transport vehicle for cholesterol that is smaller and more compact than its LDL counterpart. Unlike LDL, which deposits cholesterol in tissues, HDL removes cholesterol and transports it back to the liver. This action gives HDL a protective role in atherosclerosis, as demonstrated by the inverse relationship between HDL levels and the risk of coronary artery disease (28). However, HDL can be oxidized (primarily by HOCL), and oxidized HDL loses the ability to remove cholesterol and no longer protects against atherosclerosis (22,28).

Coronary Artery Disease

The participation of ROS in atherogenesis ensures a role in coronary artery disease, and many of the studies documenting the presence of MPO and HOCL in atheromatous plaques have involved coronary artery lesions (22). Furthermore, plasma levels of MPO show a direct correlation with the presence and severity of coronary artery disease (22,29), and in high-risk patients with chest pain, plasma MPO levels can predict the likelihood of an adverse cardiac event in the ensuing 6 months (30). Inflammatory ROS may also participate in plaque rupture (the critical event in acute myocardial infarction), because autopsy studies in humans have shown extensive staining for MPO at the site of plaque rupture (22).

Remodeling

Acute myocardial infarction is followed by a complex array of anatomical and structural changes (known as "remodeling") that alter myocardial function, and inflammatory ROS are implicated in this process (22). Laboratory mice that are bred for MPO de-

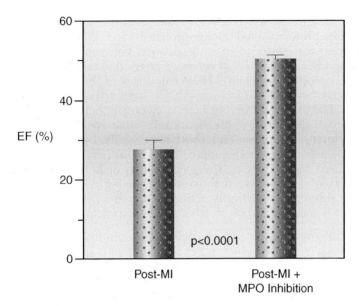

FIGURE 9.3 Left ventricular ejection fraction (EF) three weeks after acute coronary occlusion in laboratory animals treated with a myeloperoxidase (MPO) inhibitor, and in untreated control animals. Height of the bars represents mean values, and crossbars are standard errors of the mean. MI, myocardial infarction. Data from Reference 32.

ficiency (MPO-knockout mice) show much less ventricular dysfunction weeks after a myocardial infarction, when compared to control animals (31). Animal studies have also shown that daily administration of an MPO inhibitor after acute myocardial infarction is associated with improved ventricular function at 3 weeks (see Figure 9.3) (32).

Comment

The treatment of cardiovascular disease is often focused on the consequences of the disease: e.g., the treatment of congestive heart failure involves diuretics for venous congestion and systemic vasodilation to promote cardiac output, and the treatment of hypertension is aimed at lowering the blood pressure. These therapies may reduce complications from the disease, but they do not influence the disease itself. The role of inflammatory ROS in coronary artery disease, and in post infarction myocardial dysfunction, presents opportunities for antioxidant therapies that actually target the disease process. However, there has been little interest in this approach. For example, the potential benefits of MPO inhibition in coronary artery disease were recognized 15 years prior to the publication of this book (33), and the encouraging results with MPO inhibition in Figure 9.3 were published over 5 years ago, yet there is no apparent interest in evaluating MPO inhibitors in clinical trials. Attention to the potential benefits of therapy that targets oxidative stress is certainly warranted.

Sepsis

Sepsis (defined as dysregulated host response to infection that results in life-threatening organ dysfunction) is recognized as a global health problem (34), and the multiorgan dysfunction in this condition is attributed to persistent or progressive systemic inflammation (35). Several studies have shown evidence of oxidative injury in severe cases of sepsis (36-38), and the extent of oxidative injury is directly related to lethal outcomes (37), as shown in Figure 9.4. There is also evidence of antioxidant deficiency in advanced cases of sepsis (38), which magnifies the risk of oxidative tissue injury.

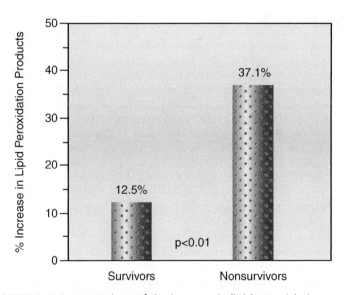

FIGURE 9.4 A comparison of the increase in lipid peroxidation products (a marker of oxidative stress) in surviving and nonsurviving ICU patients with sepsis. Data from Reference 37.

Despite a wealth of evidence implicating inflammatory ROS in sepsis-associated organ failure, there has been little enthusiasm for the use of antioxidants in this condition. Experimental studies with selected antioxidants have shown inconsistent results (39,40), but these studies have significant shortcomings. (See Chapter 12 for a discussion of these shortcomings.)

SUMMATION

As summarized in Table 9.2, reactive oxygen species (ROS) are involved in several aspects of the inflammatory response, including the beneficial effects of inflammation (i.e., microbial killing by phagocytosis) and its detrimental effects (i.e., tissue injury). The participation of ROS in inflammatory tissue injury ensures that ROS have a role in the multitude of diseases where the pathological tissue injury is attributed to inflammation (see Table 9.1). This is highlighted by the participation of ROS in two of the most dominant disease entities in modern times: cardiovascular disease and sepsis. The pivotal role of ROS in a multitude of clinical diseases creates opportunities for antioxidant therapy that have yet to be embraced.

REFERENCES

1. Turk JL. Inflammation: John Hunter's A Treatise on the Blood, Inflammation, and Gun-shot Wounds. Int J Exp Path 1994; 75:385-395.
2. Mittal M, Siddiqui MR, Tran K, et al. Reactive oxygen species in inflammation and tissue injury. Antiox Redox Signal 2014; 20:1126-1167.
3. Hurst JK, Barrette WC. Leukocyte oxygen activation and microbicidal oxidative toxins. Crit Rev Biochem Molec Biol 1989; 24:271-328.
4. Andrews S, Norton I, Salunkhe AS, et al. Control of iron metabolism in bacteria. In: Banci L, ed. Metallomics and the Cell. New York: Springer, 2013:203-239.
5. Kohanski MA, Dwyer DJ, Hayete B, et al. A common mechanism of cellular death induced by bactericidal antibiotics. Cell 2007; 130:797-810.
6. Droge W. Free radicals in the physiological control of cell function. Physiol Rev 2002; 82:47-95.
7. Winkelstein JA, Marino MC, Johnston RB et al. Chronic granulomatous disease. Report on a national registry of 368 patients. Medicine (Baltimore) 2000; 79:155-169.
8. Kuhns DB, Alvord G, Heller T, et al. Residual NADPH oxidase and survival in chronic granulomatous disease. N Engl J Med 2010; 363:2600-2610.
9. Halliwell B, Gutteridge JMC. Redox chemistry: the essentials. In: Free Radicals in Biology and Medicine. 5th ed, Oxford: Oxford University Press, 2015:30-76.

10. Montezano AC, Touyz RM. Reactive oxygen species and endothelial function – role of nitric oxide synthase uncoupling and Nox family nicotinamide adenine dinucleotide phosphate oxidases. Basic Clin Pharmacol Toxicol 2011; 110:87-94.

11. Radi R. Oxygen radicals, nitric oxide, and peroxynitrite: Redox pathways in molecular medicine. Proc Nat Acad Sci 2018; 115:5839-5848.

12. Huet O, Obata R, Aubron C, et al. Plasma-induced endothelial oxidative stress is related to the severity of septic shock. Crit Care Med 2007; 35:821-826.

13. Huet O, Cherreau C, Nicco C, et al. Pivotal role of glutathione depletion in plasma-induced endothelial oxidant stress during sepsis. Crit Care Med 2008; 36:2328-2334.

14. Chuang CY, Degendorfer G, Davies MJ. Oxidation and modification of extracellular matrix and its role in disease. Free Rad Res 2014; 48:970-989.

15. Halliwell H, Gutteridge JMC. The antioxidants in human extracellular fluids. Arch Biochem Biophys 1990; 280:1-8.

16. Smith MA, Harris PLR, Sayre LM, et al. Widespread peroxynitrite-mediated damage in Alzheimer's disease. J Neurosci 1997; 17:2653-2657.

17. Good PF, Hsu A, Werner P, et al. Protein nitration in Parkinson's disease. J Neuropath Exp Neurol 1998; 57:338-342.

18. Cai H, Chuang CY, Hawkins CL, Davies MJ. Binding of myeloperoxidase to the extracellular matrix of smooth muscle cells and subsequent matrix modification. Sci Rep 2020; 10:666.

19. Wang Z-Q, Porreca F, Cuzzocrea S, et al. A newly identified role for superoxide in inflammatory pain. J Pharmacol Exp Therap 2004; 309:869-878.

20. MacMillan-Crow LA, Cruthirds DL. Manganese superoxide dismutase in disease. Free Radic Res 2001; 34:325-326.

21. Goldblum SE, Cohen DA, Jay M, McClain CJ. Interleukin 1-induced depression of iron and zinc: Role of granulocyte and lactoferrin. Am J Physiol 1987; 252:E27-E32.

22. Ndrepepa G. Myeloperoxidase–A bridge linking inflammation and oxidative stress with cardiovascular disease. Clin Chim Acta 2019; 493:36-51.

23. Kochanek KD, Xu J, Arias E. Mortality in the United States, 2019. NCHS data brief, No. 395, December 2020. (Available at www.cdc.gov/nchs)

24. Swirski FK, Nahrendorf M. Leukocyte behavior in atherosclerosis, myocardial infarction, and heart failure. Science 2013; 339:161-166.

25. MRC/BHF Heart Protection Study of cholesterol lowering with simvastatin in 20,536 high-risk individuals: a randomized placebo-controlled trial. Lancet 2002; 360:7-22.

26. Daugherty A, Dunn JL, Rateri DL, Heinecke JW. Myeloperoxidase: a catalyst for lipoprotein oxidation, is expressed in human atherosclerotic lesions. J Clin Invest 1994; 94:437-444.

27. Steinberg D, Parthasarathy S, Carew TE, et al. Beyond cholesterol. Modifications of low-density lipoprotein that increase its atherogenicity. N Engl J Med 1989; 320:915-924.

28. Rye KA, Barter PJ. Cardioprotective functions of HDL. J Lipid Res 2014; 55:168-179.

29. Teng N, Maghzal GJ, Talib J, et al. The roles of myeloperoxidase in coronary artery disease and its potential implication in plaque rupture. Redox Report 2017; 22:51-73.

30. Brennan M-L, Penn MS, Van Lente F, et al. Prognostic value of myeloperoxidase in patients with chest pain. N Engl J Med 2003; 349:1595-1604.

31. Vasilyev N, Williams T, Brennan M-L, et al. Myeloperoxidase-generated oxidants modulate left ventricular remodeling but not infarct size after myocardial infarction. Circulation 2005; 112:2812-20.

32. Ali M, Pulli B, Courties G, et al. Myeloperoxidase inhibition improves ventricular function and remodeling after experimental myocardial infarction. JACC: Basic Trans Sci 2016; 1:633-643.

33. Malle E, Furtmuller PG, Sattler W, Obinger. Myeloperoxidase: a target for new drug development? Br J Pharmacol 2007; 152:838-854.

34. Reinhart K, Daniels R, Kissoon N, et al. Recognizing sepsis as a global health priority. N Engl J Med 2017; 377:414-417.

35. Pinsky MR, Matuschak GM. Multiple systems organ failure: failure of host defense mechanisms. Crit Care Clin 1989; 5:199–220.

36. Ware L, Fessel JP, May AK, Roberts II LJ. Plasma biomarkers of oxidant stress and development of organ failure in severe sepsis. Shock 2011; 36:12-17.

37. Motoyama T, Okamoto K, Kukita I, et al. Possible role of increased oxidant stress in multiple organ failure after systemic inflammatory response syndrome. Crit Care Med 2003; 31:1048-1052.

38. Goode HF, Cowley HC, Walker BE, et al. Decreased antioxidant status and increased lipid peroxidation in patients with septic shock and secondary organ dysfunction. Crit Care Med 1995; 23:646-651.

39. Marik PE, Khangoora V, Rivera R, et al. Hydrocortisone, vitamin C, and thiamine for the treatment of severe sepsis and septic shock: A retrospective before-after study. Chest 2017; 151:1229-1238.

40. Hwang SY, Ryoo SM, Park JE, et al. Combination therapy of vitamin C and thiamine for septic shock: a multi-centre, double-blinded randomized, controlled study. Intensive Care Med 2020; 46:2015-2025.

What does oxygen have in common with ionizing radiation?

10

"Suppose that the biological effects of exposure to nuclear radiation are no different from those of breathing oxygen."

James Lovelock (1)

At first glance, it might seem that a life-giving gas (i.e., oxygen) has little in common with the deadly emanations from the Chernobyl disaster (i.e., ionizing radiation). However, a closer look reveals a number of features that are shared by these two entities. To begin with, both are sources of energy: i.e., ionizing radiation lights the stars and powers the universe, while oxygen powers most of the life-forms on Earth. In addition, both can remove electrons from atoms or molecules (oxygen via a chemical reaction, and ionizing radiation via energy pulses), and this gives both the ability to disrupt vital cell components like membrane lipids, DNA, and cell proteins. The final feature shared by oxygen and ionizing radiation is a validation of the proposal in the introductory quote: i.e., *reactive oxygen species are primarily responsible for the damaging effects of ionizing radiation*, as is the case with oxygen. This latter feature is the principal focus of this chapter. Although this topic has a limited scope, it is included because it shines a light on the destructive nature of oxygen.

EARLY HISTORY OF RADIATION

The latter part of the 19th century was a period of intense activity in science and industry, with the introduction of the electric light, the telephone, and the automobile, along with the discovery of subatomic particles, x-rays, and radioactivity. The birth of radiation science occurred in November, 1895, when Wilhelm Röntgen discovered that cathode ray tubes could emit mysterious "X-rays" that passed through paper, cardboard, and even human flesh. Four months later (in March, 1896), the French Physicist Henri Becquerel reported that uranium salts emitted a similar type of penetrating rays, but did so spontaneously. One of Becquerel's research assistants was a recently married Polish scientist named

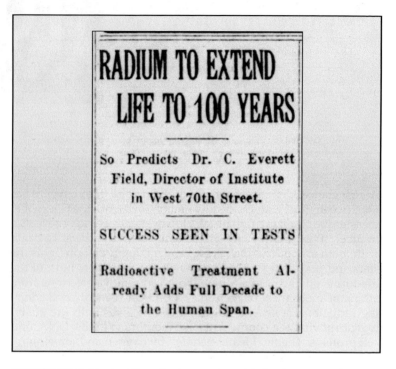

FIGURE 10.1 The heading of a front-page article in *The New York Herald* on October 14, 1921. Claims like this were responsible for radium's popularity as a miracle health aid, despite evidence of tissue injury from radium.

Marie Curie, and two years after the uranium discovery (in 1898), she and husband Pierre discovered another source of penetrating rays, radium, with a penetrating power one million times that of uranium. The Curies also observed that the penetrating rays from uranium and radium could "ionize" the surrounding air, causing it to conduct electricity. Marie Curie introduced the term *radioactivity* to describe this "ionizing radiation."

The injurious effects of ionizing radiation were experienced by both Becquerel and the Curies. Henri Becquerel developed a skin burn from a vial of radium he had carried in his vest pocket, and both Curies developed painful burn injuries on their fingers from handling radium samples. These types of burns produced painful ulcerating lesions that tended to progress rather than resolve (which is no surprise, considering that the radium isotope they were working with has a half-life of 1600 years). In recognition of radium's potential for harm, Pierre Curie included the following statement in his acceptance speech for the 1903 Nobel Prize in physics: "*It is possible to conceive that, in criminal hands, radium might prove very dangerous*" (2). (This statement would have been more prescient if Pierre had used the terms "military" or "political" instead of "criminal," although these terms are interchangeable in some instances.)

Public Misperceptions

By the turn of the 20th century, there was published evidence that exposure to radioactive elements was a source of tissue injury, and radium was being evaluated for eradicating abnormal growths on the skin. However, in the early decades of the 20th century, radium was generally perceived as a miracle substance (called "liquid sunshine") capable of curing a multitude of maladies, including old age (see Figure 10.1). In 1914, the American Medical Association included radium on its list of new therapies, and in the United States, radium was readily available in rejuvenating tonics, skin creams, soaps, and even a jockstrap (The Radio-endocrinator) for stimulating the libido. It seems unlikely that many of these products actually contained radium, since the cost of radium (in 1917) was $120,000 per gram, which is about $2.2 million today. However, a radium-enriched toothpaste available in Germany was used experimentally in the discovery of neutrons (3).

The Radium Girls

During the time of its popularity, radium was used to illuminate the numbers and dials on military instruments and watch faces. The radium was applied as a paint using slim, camel-hair brushes, and the work was done by a group of young women who became known as the "radium girls" (4). The precise application of the radium paint was aided by moistening the brush between the lips to sharpen the point. This "lip pointing" technique raised no red flags, as radium was considered safe at the time. The first sign of trouble occurred in 1921, when one of the radium girls developed unrelenting jaw pain and ulceration of the oral mucosa. The condition rapidly progressed, and within months, the entire lower jaw had become necrotic and abscessed. Necrotic pieces of mandible began to appear in her mouth, and the entire mandible was removed in this fashion, without surgery. Consultation with numerous dentists and physicians failed to produce a definitive diagnosis. Eleven months after the condition first appeared, the necrosis in the lower jaw eroded into the internal jugular vein, and the 24-year-old radium girl died from exsanguination into her mouth.

By 1925, as many as 50 radium girls had developed a similar condition, and a report was published in that year that implicated radium as the cause of this condition. However this received little attention, and radium continued to be readily available for public consumption. Predictably, it took the death of a prominent member of society to sound the alarm. A steel magnate named Eben Byers had ingested thousands of bottles of a radioactive tonic (Radiothor), as prescribed by his physician, and he developed aggressive jaw necrosis and died (in 1931). Shortly after his high-profile death, the Federal Trade Commission put a "cease and desist" order against the Radiothor tonic, and this heralded the downfall of the radium industry. It took another 6 years for a government agency to officially recognize that the radium girls were victims of radium exposure in the workplace. Most of the them had died by this time, but their story sparked the emergence of the Occupational Safety and Health Administration.

Comment

The historical account just presented is not meant only as an interesting aside, but is included because the persistent lack of awareness and disregard for the harmful effects of radiation (which lasted 30-40 years) is not very different from the current state of affairs with oxygen. The general public is clearly unaware of the hazards of oxygen, even though they voraciously ingest antioxidants, and would not be without cellophane wrapping and tightly sealed plastic containers that shield food from the damaging effects of oxygen. As for the medical community, the disregard for oxygen toxicity is provided by a survey of more than 100,000 arterial blood gas samples from patients receiving supplemental oxygen, which showed that arterial PO_2 levels were excessively high in 75% of the samples (5).

SHARED MECHANISMS

Like oxygen, ionizing radiation dislodges electrons from molecules, which creates the ability to disrupt and damage vital cell components (i.e., membrane lipids, DNA, and cell proteins). Damage to the DNA molecule has been the principal focus of

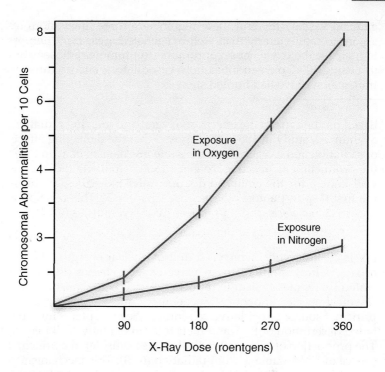

FIGURE 10.2 Effects of increasing doses of X-irradiation on chromosomal abnormalities in spiderwort microspores exposed to radiation in the presence and absence of oxygen. Data from Reference 7.

studies on radiation injury, and this damage is very similar to the damage associated with oxidative stress (which is described in Chapter 8). One exception is the tendency for radiation damage to occur in clusters, which is more difficult to repair (6).

Oxygen as a Radiosensitizer

Early observations revealed that radiation-induced DNA damage was much greater in the presence of oxygen. This is demonstrated in Figure 10.2, which shows the effects of X-irradiation on chromosomal aberrations in plant microspores in the presence and absence of oxygen (7). This "radiosensitizing" effect of oxygen plays an important role in the efficacy of radiotherapy for the treatment of malignant tumors. The growth of tumors is typically accompanied by areas of ischemia within the tumor mass from disorganized vascularity, and these regions are three times more resistant to radiotherapy than well-oxygenated areas (8). Attempts to increase the oxygenation of tumors (to promote radiosensitivity) using 100% oxygen inhalation, vasodilators, and erythrocyte transfusions have had limited success.

Reactive Oxygen Species

Based on the synergistic effects of oxygen and ionizing radiation, a landmark study in 1954 (9) proposed that the damaging effects of radiation and oxygen share the same mechanism of action: i.e., the production of "reactive oxygen species." Ionizing radiation is well-known for the ability to disrupt water molecules, as this is the first step in photosynthesis. (See Chapter 7.) This reaction is known as *radiolysis*, and it produces hydroxyl radicals (OH·); i.e.,

$$H_2O + eV \rightarrow H^+ + e^- + OH^·$$ (10.1)

(eV is electron volts, which is a unit of nuclear energy). The hydroxyl radical is one of the reactive oxygen species (ROS) generated by O_2 metabolism in mitochondria. It is the most reactive chemical species known in biochemistry and is considered the principal source of oxidative cell injury. (See Chapter 8 for a detailed description of ROS and their roles in oxidative cell injury.) The production of hydroxyl radicals is also considered a principal source of DNA damage from radiation (6,10). This mechanism is more likely than direct DNA damage because water is the major constituent of cells and is the most abundant target for radiation.

In an aerobic environment at physiological pH, radiolysis also produces hydrogen peroxide and superoxide radicals (10), which means that radiation can initiate a reaction sequence that is the reverse of O_2 metabolism. This is illustrated in Figure 10.3 (11), which shows that *the production of ROS is a shared mechanism for the damaging effects of both ionizing radiation and oxygen*. The ability of ionizing radiation to generate ROS is demonstrated by the following example (10): a 3.2 MeV pulse of alpha particles generates about 2,000 ROS, which corresponds to an ROS concentration of about 19 nM in the cell nucleus; a concentration expected to produce extensive oxidative damage. The production of ROS would also explain why irradiated cells are often accompanied by damage in surrounding "bystander" cells (10), since radiation-generated hydrogen peroxide can move freely from cell to cell.

The Cost of Breathing Air

The presence of oxidized DNA fragments in the urine of healthy subjects indicates that there is a low level of oxidative DNA damage during normal aerobic metabolism. Measuring the urinary excretion of these oxidized residues allows an estimation of the number of oxidation "hits" to the DNA molecule each day—in one study, this amounted to 5×10^{15} DNA hits per day for an average-sized adult (12). The radiation dose needed to produce a similar number of oxidation hits to DNA has been estimated at 1,000 millisieverts (mSv) per year (1). To place this radiation dose in perspective, Table 10.1 shows the average radiation dose associated with some common radiographic procedures, along with the annual dose of radiation that is considered safe. Note that a dose of 1,000 mSv is equivalent to 10,000 chest x-rays, and it is 20 times higher than the recommended safe limit of radiation exposure. This means that *breathing atmospheric oxygen for one year is equivalent to the radiation exposure from 10,000 chest x-rays!*

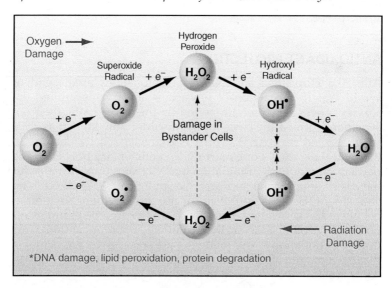

FIGURE 10.3 The participation of reactive oxygen species in the damaging effects of oxygen and ionizing radiation. Adapted from Reference 11. See text for further explanation.

Table 10.1	Selected Radiation Doses
Condition	**Radiation Dose**
Chest x-ray	0.1 mSv
Head CT	2 mSv
Head CT with contrast	4 mSv
CT angiography (chest)	10 mSv
Safe dose for 1 year[†]	≤50 mSv
Breathing air for 1 year[*]	1,000 mSv

[†]From the Environmental Protection Agency (epa.gov).
[*]See text for explanation. mSv = millisieverts.

ANTIOXIDANT PROTECTION

After the Hiroshima and Nagasaki detonations at the end of World War II, a coalition of physicians and nurses studied the survivors over a two-month period (in the fall of 1945); their observations formed the basis for the disorder now known as *acute radiation syndrome* (ARS), which is characterized by damage in the central nervous, bone marrow, and alimentary tract (13). The participation of ROS in radiation injury creates opportunities for the use of antioxidants to prevent or mitigate ARS. Although no antioxidant has been approved for use in ARS, there are a number of studies showing that antioxidants can provide radioprotection, and oncologists typically recommend avoiding antioxidants during radiotherapy. The following are some of the antioxidants that have proven effective in curtailing radiation injury. (Antioxidants are described in detail in Chapter 12.)

Glutathione

Early studies showed that ionizing radiation inhibited the activity of proteins with sulfhydryl (SH) groups (14), and one of these proteins is glutathione, a tripeptide that serves as a major intracellular antioxidant. These studies prompted an evaluation of glutathione as a radioprotective agent, and the results are shown in Figure 10.4 (15). In this case, laboratory mice exposed to increasing doses of X-irradiation showed a decrease in mortality rate if they were pretreated with glutathione (given as a single dose subcutaneously, just prior to radiation exposure). Despite promising results like this, the exogenous administration of glutathione is problematic. (These problems are described in Chapter 12.) However, there are two alternatives to glutathione. One of these is N-acetylcysteine, a glutathione surrogate that has been used successfully for glutathione replacement in acetaminophen overdoses. The other alternative is described next.

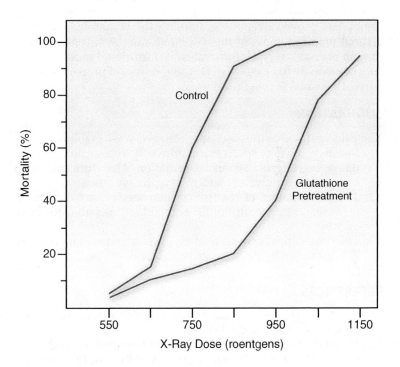

FIGURE 10.4 Mortality rate at 28 days following exposure to increasing doses of X-irradiation in laboratory mice and the effect of pretreatment with the antioxidant glutathione (4 mg/g given subcutaneously just prior to irradiation). Data from Reference 15.

Amifostine

Amifostine is a prodrug that is converted to a sulfhydryl-containing antioxidant (like glutathione) in the vascular endothelium. This antioxidant is unique because it provides radioprotection in normal tissues, but not in neoplastic tissue (probably because of dysfunctional vascularity in neoplasms) (16), and this makes it well-suited for protecting normal tissues of the host during radiotherapy. At the present time, amifostine is approved for use in ameliorating xerostomia in patients undergoing radiotherapy for head and neck cancer.

Vitamin E

Vitamin E is a family of eight naturally occurring isoforms that serve as lipid-soluble antioxidants. One of the isoforms, γ-tocotrienol, has proven effective in limiting the hematologic and intestinal manifestations of the acute radiation syndrome in non-human primates (17). Unfortunately, γ-tocotrienol must be given subcutaneously to be effective (18), and only oral preparations are currently available for clinical use.

SUMMATION

The principal points in this chapter can be stated as follows:
1. Reactive oxygen species are primarily responsible for the damaging effects of ionizing radiation. Therefore, radiation injury can be viewed as a form of oxidative stress.
2. The participation of reactive oxygen species in radiation injury creates opportunities for antioxidants as radioprotective agents.
3. The similarities between oxidative injury and radiation injury is a testament to the destructive nature of oxygen.

REFERENCES

1. Lovelock J. The Ages of Gaia: A Biography of Our Living Earth. New York: W.W. Norton & Co, 1995:165.
2. Mould RF. Pierre Curie, 1859-1906. Curr Oncol 2007; 14:74-82.
3. Bodanis D. E=mc^2: A Biography of the World's Most Famous Equation. New York: Berkley Books, 2001:96.
4. Moore K. Radium Girls. The Dark Story of America's Shining Women. Naperville, IL: Sourcebooks, Inc, 2017.

5. Helmerhorst HJF, Schultz MJ, van der Voort PHJ, et al. Self-reported attitudes versus actual practice of oxygen therapy by ICU physicians and nurses. Ann Intensive Care 2014; 4:23.

6. O'Neill P, Wardman P. Radiation chemistry comes before radiation biology. In J Radiat Biol 2009; 85:9-25.

7. Giles NH, Riley HP. The effect of oxygen on the frequency of X-ray induced chromosomal rearrangements in Tradescantia microspores. Proc Natl Acad Sci 1949; 35:640-646.

8. Rockwell S, Dobrucki IT, Kim EY, et al. Hypoxia and radiation therapy: Past history, ongoing research, and future promise. Curr Mol Med 2009; 9:442-458.

9. Gerschamn R, Gilbert DL, Nye SW, et al. Oxygen poisoning and x-irradiation, a mechanism in common. Science 1954; 119:623-626.

10. Azzam EI, Jay-Gerin J-P, Pain D. Ionizing radiation-induced metabolic oxidative stress and prolonged cell injury. Cancer Lett 2012; 327:48-60.

11. Lane N. Oxygen: The Molecule That Made The World. Oxford: Oxford University Press, 2002:112.

12. Shigenaga MK, Gimeno CJ, Ames BN. Urinary 8-hydroxy-2′-deoxyguanosine as a biological marker of in vivo oxidative DNA damage. Proc Natl Acad Sci 1989; 86:9697-9701.

13. Finch SC. Acute radiation syndrome. JAMA 1987; 258:664-667.

14. Barron ESG, Dickman SR. Studies on the mechanism of action of ionizing radiations. II. Inhibition of sulfhydryl enzymes by alpha, beta, and gamma rays. J Gen Physiol 1949; 32:595-605.

15. Chapman WH, Cronkite EP. Further studies of the beneficial effect of glutathione on X-irradiated mice. Proc Soc Exp Biol Med 1950; 75:318-322.

16. Kouvaris JR, Kouloulias VE, Vlahos L. Amifostine: the first selective-target and broad-spectrum radioprotector. Oncologist 2007; 12:738-747.

17. Singh VK, Kulkami S, Fatanmi OO, et al. Radioprotective efficacy of gamma-tocotrienol in nonhuman primates. Radiat Res 2016; 185:285-298.

18. Singh VK, Hauer-Jensen M. γ-tocotrienol as a promising countermeasure for acute radiation syndrome: current status. Int J Molec Sci 2016; 17:663.

Does oxygen promote aging?

11

"All human things are subject to decay."

John Dryden (a)

The relentless march of aging is a complex and multifaceted phenomenon that includes loss of functionality, impaired recovery from acute illness or physiological stress, and an increased risk of age-related diseases (e.g., atherosclerosis). At the cellular level, aging involves aberrations in the DNA molecule that trigger loss of the ability for cell replication. Oxidative stress promotes aging at the cellular level, and also plays an important role in age-related diseases. The following is a brief summary of aging, and the contributions of oxygen and its more reactive offspring.

CELLULAR BASIS OF AGING

In the adult human, as many as 70,000,000,000 (70 billion) cells die each day by a gene-regulated process known as *apoptosis* (1). This process is triggered by a regulator gene that activates a protein known as *p53* (the number refers to the molecular mass of the protein). The activated p53 protein can disrupt mitochondrial membranes to release cytochrome C into the cytoplasm, and this activates a family of proteases known as *caspases* that rapidly degrade all vital cell components (2). The resulting cell disruption does not incite an inflammatory response, which is a feature that distinguishes apoptosis from "necrosis" (traumatic cell death).

Cell Senescence

The cells that are lost by apoptosis must be replaced to preserve the mass and function of vital organs. This replacement is accomplished by the process of *cell replication*, where cells duplicate their DNA and divide to form an identical replica of the parent cell. However, there is a limit to the number of times cells can replicate (typically 50 – 70 times). This is known as the *Hayflick limit*, named after the American anatomist, Leonard Hayflick, who first reported this phenomenon in 1961 (3). When the Hayflick limit

149

is reached, cell replication ceases permanently, and cells enter a state of *replicative senescence* (4). Senescent cells have two characteristics that contribute to aging. First, they are resistant to apoptosis and have been described as "cancer cells that don't divide" (5). Second, they secrete proinflammatory mediators that generate a chronic, low-grade inflammation, and this is the driving force for age-related diseases like atherosclerosis (6) and osteoarthritis (7). This type of age-related inflammation has been given the silly name of *inflammaging* (8).

Telomeres

The senescence that occurs after cells have reached their replicative (Hayflick) limit is attributed to the shortening of *telomeres*, which are repetitive sequences of nucleotide bases that serve as a protective covering on the end of chromosomes (like the plastic aglets that protect the ends of shoelaces) (9). The telomerase enzyme that synthesizes telomeres is active only during gestation. As a result, repeated cell replications after birth results in progressive shortening of telomeres, and this eventually exposes the unprotected ends of chromosomes and triggers a *DNA damage response* that culminates in the arrest of cell replication. This response, which is illustrated in Figure 11.1, involves activation of the same p53 protein involved in apoptosis, but in this case, the activated protein triggers a signaling pathway that results in cell senescence.

The DNA damage response can be triggered by any aberration in the DNA molecule that cannot be repaired, and it is a mechanism for preventing the replication of genetically defective cells. A dysfunctional DNA damage response can lead to unconstrained cell replication, which is the hallmark of neoplastic growth.

Senotherapy

The importance of cell senescence in the aging process has created a new approach to aging called *senotherapeutics*, which includes *senolytic agents* that eliminate senescent cells by promoting apoptosis, and *senomorphic agents* that suppress the inflammatory response to cell senescence (5,10).

Senolytic Agents

Senescent cells express a protein that blocks apoptosis, and agents that inactivate this protein make up the first generation of senolytic agents. Most are repurposed chemotherapeutic agents, although one commonly used drug, aspirin, has documented seno-

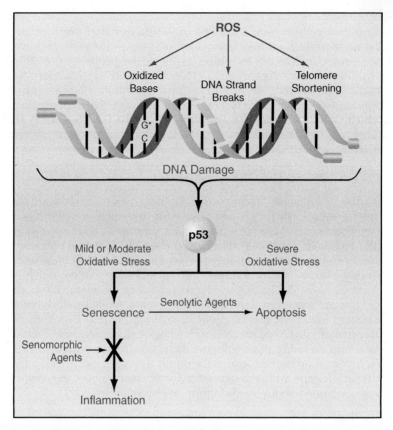

FIGURE 11.1 Diagram showing the pathways involved in the contribution of reactive oxygen species (ROS) to aging and age-related diseases. The asterisk indicates that guanine is especialy suceptible to oxidative modification. See text for explanation.

lytic effects (11). Senolytic therapy in animal models of aging has been promising, with evidence of increased longevity, reduced frailty, and slowing of age-related cognitive decline (4,5,10). As a result of these studies, there are currently (in 2021) at least 12 human trials of senolytic therapy for age-related diseases (5). Most are ongoing, but the preliminary results of one trial shows that senolytic therapy reduces the burden of senescent cells in patients with diabetic nephropathy (12).

Senomorphic Agents

Senescent cells secrete a variety of substances that promote inflammation (e.g.,interleukins, chemokines, proteases), and senomorphic agents act to inhibit or block the production of this proinflammatory "secretome." The most studied senomorphic agent is rapamycin, an immunosuppressant that inhibits a protein kinase known as mTOR (mammalian target of rapamycin), which is the "engine" for the proinflammatory secretome (13). (This mTOR is also involved in the longevity effect of calorie restriction, as explained later.)

FREE RADICAL THEORY OF AGING

Studies of longevity in different animal species have revealed an inverse relationship between maximum life span and the basal metabolic rate (BMR) per unit of mass (known as the "mass-specific metabolic rate") (14). The higher the BMR (per unit of mass), the shorter the life span of the species. This relationship is demonstrated by comparing the life span of laboratory mice and humans: i.e., lab mice have a resting metabolic rate of about 220 kcal/kg/day and a maximum life span of 3-4 years, while humans have a resting metabolic rate of about 20 kcal/kg/day and a maximum life span of 110-120 years. (*Note:* The longest documented life span for a human is 122 years and 164 days, which was achieved by a French woman named Jeanne Calment, who died in 1997 (15). Of interest, Jeanne smoked cigarettes for 96 years, never exercised, and consumed about one kilogram of chocolate weekly!)

The negative influence of metabolic rate on longevity suggests that one or more products of metabolism contributes to aging, and a landmark article published in 1956 proposed that reactive oxygen species (ROS) are the age-promoting metabolites (16). The author of this article was a chemist (and recent medical school graduate) named Denham Harman, who had worked for the Shell Oil Company studying free radical reactions in petroleum products. He proposed that aging is a gradual decline in cell function caused by cumulative damage from ROS generated by aerobic metabolism. This is known as the *free radical theory of aging* (a misnomer, since ROS are not always free radicals), and it represents the first mention of the destructive potential of oxygen and its congeners in the medical literature.

Mechanisms

Reactive oxygen species (ROS) have three actions that can trigger a DNA damage response and thereby promote the cellular processes involved in aging (17-19). These actions are depicted in Figure 11.1 and include DNA strand breaks, oxidative modification of nucleotide bases (particularly guanine), and telomere shortening. During normal metabolism, these actions probably have little consequence (due to DNA repair mechanisms), although there is evidence that oxidative DNA damage increases with aging (19). However, during conditions of heightened ROS activity (i.e., oxidative stress), the DNA damage from ROS can trigger either cell senescence or apoptosis. The p53 protein regulates the response to oxidative stress (20). When the oxidative stress is mild or moderate, the p53 protein activates cell senescence, while during periods of extreme oxidative stress (e.g., from radiation), the p53 protein initiates apoptosis, which removes cells that are severely damaged.

Table 11.1 Age-Related Diseases that Involve Oxidative Stress

Organ System	Diseases
Brain	Alzheimer Disease Parkinson Disease
Eye	Cataracts Macular Degeneration
Cardiovascular	Atherosclerosis Hypertension Ischemic Stroke Coronary Artery Disease Renovascular Disease
Lungs	COPD
Endocrine	Diabetes (Type II) Diabetic Microangiopathy Obesity
Bone and Joint	Osteoporosis Osteoarthritis

Age-Related Diseases

In addition to promoting aging on a cellular level, oxidative stress also promotes age-related diseases because chronic, low-grade inflammation plays an important role in many of these diseases, and ROS are a key ingredient in the inflammatory response, as described in Chapter 9.

Some of the age-related diseases that are linked to oxidative stress are listed in Table 11.1. (See Chapter 9 for a description of how ROS participate in cardiovascular disease.)

Comment

Despite a wealth of evidence indicating that oxidative stress contributes to aging, the free radical theory of aging has fallen out of favor in recent years. This is primarily due to studies showing that antioxidant therapy does not reliably curtail the progression of age-related diseases (21,22). However, there are several problems with the studies of antioxidant therapy performed to date, including inappropriate antioxidant selection, inadequate treatment periods (i.e., effects on age-related diseases may take several years to bear fruit), lack of guidelines about appropriate dosing, and limitations in the bioavailability of some exogenously administered antioxidants. The failure of antioxidant therapy should not negate the importance of oxidative stress in aging, just as our lack of effective therapy for many diseases does not negate the presence of the disease.

The free radical theory of aging does, however, require an amendment. The original theory proposed that the culprit in aging was the accumulated damage from the everyday production of ROS during "normal" metabolism. However, the contribution of ROS to aging is more likely to occur during periods of intense ROS activity (i.e., oxidative stress), as occurs with acute illnesses (e.g., infections), physical traumas, toxic drug and alcohol ingestions, physiological stress (e.g., sleep deprivation, strenuous exercise), and even psychological stress (e.g., anxiety).

CALORIE RESTRICTION

The apparent negative influence of the metabolic rate on longevity (mentioned earlier) created interest in restricting the intake of nutritional calories as an antiaging strategy. Subsequent studies in animals has provided convincing evidence that a decrease in the daily intake of calories (usually by 40%) can increase the life span and impede the progression of age-related diseases (23-25). The longevity benefits of calorie restriction have been reported mostly in laboratory mice, but they have also been documented in rhesus monkeys, fish, nematodes, fruit flies, and even yeast organisms (24). In laboratory mice, a 40% reduction in daily caloric intake is associated with a 50-60% increase in life span (19,25). Studies of longevity extension in humans are not available (and are difficult to conduct), but there is evidence that long-term calorie restriction (for at least 3 years) in middle-aged subjects is accompanied by a considerable decrease in the risk of age-related diseases like atherosclerosis (26).

Mechanisms

The longevity benefit of calorie restriction is associated with a decrease in oxidative DNA damage, as shown in Figure 11.2 (19). This observation adds credence to the role of oxidative stress in aging (27). However, the calorie restriction story is much more complex; i.e., the principal mechanism for the longevity benefit

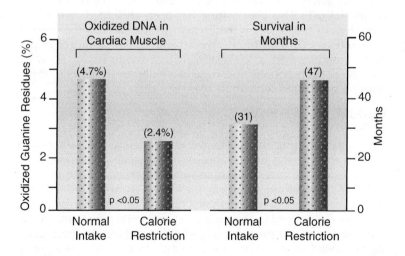

FIGURE 11.2 The effects of a 40% reduction in daily caloric intake on oxidized DNA in cardiac muscle, and survival, in laboratory mice. Oxidized DNA represents the concentration of oxidized guanine residues in cardiac muscle at 24 months, expressed in relation to a standard concentration of native guanine. All data points represent mean values. Data from Reference 19.

of calorie restriction is activation of a family of proteins known as *sirtuins* (28). There are seven sirtuins in mammals, and they have a variety of longevity-promoting actions, including transcriptional silencing of genes involved in aging, enhanced DNA repair, delayed cell senescence, and inhibition of mitochondrial ROS production (28,29). Thus, the longevity-promoting effects of calorie restriction are not the sole result of a decrease in oxidative stress.

The discovery of sirtuins has led to a search for chemical substances that can activate sirtuins and mimic the longevity benefit of calorie restriction. The most potent sirtuin activator discovered to date is *resveratrol* (30), a natural polyphenol found in the skins of grapes, blueberries, and raspberries. Resveratrol has shown a longevity benefit in laboratory mice maintained on a high-calorie diet (thereby mimicking the effect of calorie restriction) (31). In addition, resveratrol alters β-amyloid deposition in the brain in a manner that would benefit patients with Alzheimer disease (32).

The French Paradox

The longevity benefit of resveratrol might also explain the French paradox, which refers to the relatively low mortality rate from coronary artery disease in France, despite a diet that is rich in saturated fat (33). This observation has been attributed to the consumption of red wine by the French, which exceeds that of other countries (33). This implicates resveratrol as the source of this phenomenon, which is consistent with a recent report showing that the consumption of red wine in moderate amounts (200 mL daily) is associated with an increase in sirtuin levels (34).

MAXIMUM LIFE SPAN

The negative influence of oxygen on longevity can be inferred from a comparison of the maximum life span of air-breathing creatures (i.e., oxygen consumers) and trees (i.e., oxygen producers). For air-breathing creatures, the longest documented life span is 211 years in a bowhead whale (35). In comparison, the oldest living tree on record is a Great Basin bristlecone pine in the White Mountains of California , which is 5,062 years old, and the oldest clonal colony of trees (i.e., share a single root system) is a group of quaking aspen trees in the Fishlake National Forest in Utah, which are estimated to be 80,000 years old (36).

SUMMATION

The following points in this chapter deserve emphasis.

There is considerable evidence to indicate that reactive oxygen species (ROS) are intimately involved in the aging process. The major contribution of ROS to aging is not from ROS production during normal, everyday metabolism (as proposed in the free radical theory of aging), but rather from periods of heightened ROS activity, i.e., oxidative stress.

Oxidative stress has several effects that can promote aging at the cellular level, including accelerated telomere shortening, DNA damage from strand breakage, and oxidative modification of nucleotide bases. Each of these aberrations can trigger a "DNA damage response" that results in either cell death (apoptosis) or the arrest of cell replication (cell senescence).

Oxidative stress also participates in age-related diseases because the driving force for these conditions is a chronic low-grade inflammation that is triggered by the accumulation of senescent cells. The pivotal role of oxidative stress in inflammation (described in Chapter 9) thus ensures their role in the pathophysiology of age-related diseases.

Finally, the importance of oxidative stress in aging has been downgraded because of studies showing that antioxidant therapy does not reliably alter the coarse of age-related diseases. However, antioxidant studies have major shortcomings (e.g., limited bioavailability of exogenous antioxidants), and failure of antioxidant therapy should not negate the importance of oxidative stress in aging, just as our lack of effective therapy for many diseases does not negate the presence of the disease.

REFERENCES

a. Dryden J. Mac Flecknoe, 1682. (First line of the poem.)

1. Divan A, Royds JA. Molecular Biology: A Very Short Introduction. Oxford: Oxford University Press, 2016: 75.
2. Alberts B, Johnson A, Lewis J, et al, (eds). Molecular Biology of the Cell, 6th ed. New York: Garland Science, 2015:1014-1034.
3. Hayflick L, Moorhead PS. The serial cultivation of human diploid cell strains. Exp Cell Res 1961; 25:585-561.
4. Kirkland JL, Tchkonia T. Cellular senescence: a translational perspective. EBioMedicine 2017; 21:21-28.
5. Robbins PD, Jurk D, Khosla S, et al. Senolytic drugs: Reducing senescent cell viability to extend health span. Annu Rev Pharmacol Toxicol 2021; 61:779-803.

6. Childs BG, Baker DJ, Wijshake T, et al. Senescent intimal foam cells are deleterious at all stages of atherosclerosis. Science 2016; 354:472-477.

7. Jeon OH, Kim C, Laberge R-M, et al. Local clearance of senescent cells attenuates the development of post-traumatic osteoarthritis and creates a pro-regenerative environment. Nat Med 2017; 23:775-781.

8. Francheschi F, Garagnani P, Vitale G, et al. Inflammaging and "garb-aging'. Trends Endocrinol Metab 2017; 28:199-212.

9. Shay JW. Telomeres and ageing. Curr Opin Cell Biol 2018; 52:1-7.

10. Shetty AK, Kodali M, Upadhya R, Madhu LN. Emerging anti-aging strategies – scientific basis and efficacy. Aging Dis 2018; 9:1165-1184.

11. Feng M, Kim J, Field K, et al. Aspirin ameliorates the long-term adverse effects of doxorubicin through suppression of cellular senescence. FASEB Bioadv 2019; 1:579-590.

12. Hickson LJ, Langhi Prata LGP, Bobart SA, et al. Senolytics decrease senescent cells in humans: preliminary report from a clinical trial of dasatinib plus quercetin in individuals with diabetic kidney disease. EBioMedicine 2019; 47:446-456.

13. Laberge R-M, Sun Y, Orjalo AV, et al. MTOR regulates the pro-tumorigenic senescence-associated secretory phenotype by promoting IL-1A translation. Nat Cell Biol 2015; 17:1049-1061.

14. Pearl R. The Rate of Living: Being an Account of Some Experimental Studies on the Biology of Life Duration. New York: A.A. Knopf, 1928.

15. West G. Scale. The Universal Laws of Life, Growth, and Death in Organisms, Cities, and Companies. New York: Penguin Books, 2017:177-189

16. Harman D. Aging: a theory based on free radical and radiation chemistry. J Gerontol 1956; 11:298-300.

17. Jan HJ, Hoeijmakers. DNA damage, aging, and cancer. New Engl J Med 2009; 361:1475-1485.

18. von Zglinicki T. Oxidative stress shortens telomeres. Trends Biochem Sci 2002; 27:339-344.

19. Hamilton ML, Van Remmen H, Drake JA, et al. Does oxidative damage to DNA increase with age? PNAS 2001; 98:10469-10474.

20. Beyfuss K, Hood DA. A systematic review of p53 regulation of oxidative stress in skeletal muscle. Redox Report 2018; 23:100-117.

21. da Costa JP, Vitorino R, Silva GM, et al. A synopsis on aging – theories, mechanisms, and future prospects. Ageing Res Rev 2016; 29:90-112.

22. Sadowska-Bartosz I, Bartosz G. Effect of antioxidants on aging and longevity. BioMed Res Internat 2014; Article ID 404680:1-17.

23. Sohal RS, Weindruch R. Oxidative stress, calorie restriction, and aging. Science 1996; 273:59-63.

24. Fontana L, Partridge L, Longo VD. Extending healthy life span – from yeast to humans. Science 2010; 328:321-326.

25. Walford RL. Maximum Life Span. New York: W.W. Norton & Co, 1983:98-113.

26. Fontana L, Meyer TE, Klein S, Holloszy JO. Long-term calorie restriction is highly effective in reducing the risk of atherosclerosis in humans. Proc Nat Acad Sci 2004; 101:6659-6663.

27. Gredilla R, Barja G. Minireview: the role of oxidative stress in relation to caloric restriction and longevity. Endocrinology 2005; 146:3713-3717.

28. Guarente L. Sirtuins, aging, and medicine. N Engl J Med 2011; 364:2235-2244.

29. Lee S-H, Lee J-H, Lee H-Y, Min K-J. Sirtuin signaling in cellular senescence and aging. BMB Rep 2019; 52:24-34.

30. Milne JC, Denu JM. The Sirtuin family: therapeutic targets to treat diseases of aging. Curr Opin Chem Biol 2008; 12:11-17.

31. Bauer JA, Pearson KJ, Price NL, et al. Resveratrol improves health and survival of mice on a high-calorie diet. Nature 2006; 444:337-342.

32. Pasinetti GM, Wang J, Ho L, et al. Roles of resveratrol and other grape-derived polyphenols in Alzheimer's disease prevention and treatment. Biochim Biophys Acta 2015; 1852:1202-1208.

33. Renaud S, de Lorgeril M. Wine, alcohol, platelets, and the French paradox. Lancet 1992 for coronary artery disease. Lancet 1992; 339:1523-1526.

34. Gambini J, Gimeno-Mallench L, Olaso-Gonzalez G, et al. Moderate red wine consumption increases the expression of longevity-associated genes in controlled human populations and extends lifespan in *Drosophila melanogaster*. Antiox 2021; 10:301.

35. www.futurelearn.com. Accessed 5/31/2021

36. www.livescience.com. Accessed 4/6/2019

Why do our bodies decompose after we die?

12

"Absence of evidence is not evidence of absence."

Carl Sagan (*a*)

We are continuously bathed in a gas (oxygen) that is relentless in its pursuit to dismantle organic life-forms. (For evidence of this, peel and slice a potato, and leave the potato slices exposed to air. You will notice that the potato begins to turn brown after just a few minutes, which is caused by oxidation of the starches in the potato.) The moment we die, the dismantling power of oxygen begins in earnest, and our bodies begin to decompose. The earliest sign of this is the fetid odor of death, a manifestation of the oxidative breakdown of our polyunsaturated fatty acids, which is the same process (known as "rancidity") that produces the foul odor in decaying food.

Humans have two attributes that keep oxygen (oxidation) at bay during our lifetime. The first one is our aqueous interior, which serves as a protective shield against the intrusion of oxygen (see Chapter 3). The second attribute (the one that stops working when we die) is a virtual army of enzymes, vitamins, and reducing agents that are dedicated to fighting oxidation. These chemical species are called "antioxidants," and their job is to delay, prevent, or remove oxidative damage from our midst (1). This chapter is an introduction to some of the most studied antioxidants, including what they do and what happens when they are depleted or deficient.

Caveat: It is important to emphasize that this chapter is only a cursory introduction to the topic of antioxidant protection, and will not describe the entirety of endogenous antioxidants. This would require volumes of text, along with frequent revisions. (The scope of this topic is demonstrated by a recent PubMed search on antioxidants that yielded 150,000 citations from the past 5 years; an average of 30,000 citations yearly.)

ANTIOXIDANT CHEMISTRY

The human body is equipped with a robust system of antioxidant protection that includes a variety of protective methods, and a wider variety of chemical species (antioxidants) that can execute these methods. The major components of this system are listed in Table 12.1. The following is a description of the principal, or most studied, endogenous antioxidants.

Superoxide Dismutase

In 1968, two members of the Biochemistry Department at Duke University (Joe McCord and Irwin Fridovich) discovered an enzyme in human erythrocytes that catalyzed the following reaction (2):

$$2O_2^{\cdot} + 2H^+ \rightarrow H_2O_2 + O_2 \qquad (12.1)$$

where $O_2^{\cdot}$ is the superoxide radical, and H_2O_2 is hydrogen peroxide. This is a "dismutation" reaction (i.e., a reaction in which the same chemical species is both oxidized and reduced); hence, the enzyme was named *superoxide dismutase* (SOD). The Duke investigators also discovered that this enzyme could block the oxidation of epinephrine to adrenochrome, which is mediated by superoxide radicals. This was the first evidence of an endogenous substance that could inhibit biological oxidation, i.e., an antioxidant. The discovery of superoxide dismutase is considered the foundation for what we know today about oxidative stress, and it has been cited as the most important discovery in modern biology that has not been awarded a Nobel Prize (3).

The superoxide dismutase (SOD) enzymes are metalloproteins that use transition metals to carry out the combined oxidation and reduction reactions that they catalyze. The SOD in mitochondria uses manganese (Mn-SOD), while the SOD in the cytoplasm and extracellular fluid has copper and zinc in its active site (Cu/Zn-SOD). The dismutation reaction proceeds without SOD, but in the presence of the enzyme, the reaction is instantaneous (1).

Antioxidant Actions

The role of SOD as an antioxidant is based on the ability to clear superoxide radicals (see Figure 12.1). The importance of this role is shown in studies involving genetic manipulation in laboratory mice. Animals that are bred to be deficient in Mn-SOD survive only a few weeks and exhibit severe degenerative changes in the heart and brain (4), while animals that express increased levels of Cu/Zn-SOD are resistant to oxidative lung damage (5).

TABLE 12.1 The Robust System of Antioxidant Protection

Method	Antioxidants
Remove Superoxide Radicals	Superoxide dismutase
Remove Hydrogen Peroxide	Glutathione peroxidase, glutathione, selenium*, peroxiredoxins, thioredoxin, catalase
Inhibit Lipid Peroxidation	α-tocopherol, ubiquinol, urate
Reduce Iron Availability	Transferrin, lactoferrin, ferritin, ceruloplasmin, hemopexin, haptoglobin
Inactivate (Scavenge) ROS	Albumin, ascorbate, α-tocopherol, β-carotene, bilirubin, glutathione, lipoic acid, peroxiredoxins, pyruvate, thioredoxin, urate
Regenerate Antioxidants	Ascorbate, glutathione, glutathione reductase, lipoic acid, thioredoxin reductase, thiamine*, ubiquinol

*Indirect effect. ROS = reactive oxygen species.

The efficacy of SOD as an exogenous antioxidant is limited by a very short half-life in the bloodstream (about 8 seconds) and difficulty crossing cell membranes. Both shortcomings are mitigated by the delivery of SOD in liposomes (6), but commercial preparations are not available. There has been a prolonged (30-year) effort to develop effective "SOD mimetics" for clinical use, but these have suffered from a limited specificity of action (7). A final problem with use of SOD as an antioxidant is the expected increase in production of hydrogen peroxide, since this can actually promote oxidative injury if the mechanisms for clearing hydrogen peroxide (described next) are impaired or deficient.

The Glutathione Redox System

One of the principal mechanisms for protection against oxidative cell injury is to reduce hydrogen peroxide directly to water, which bypasses the production of highly destructive hydroxyl radicals. (See Chapter 8 for a description of how hydrogen peroxide promotes oxidative cell injury.) A number of enzymes can facilitate this reaction (see Table 12.1), but the most effective of these is *glutathione peroxidase*, which reduces hydrogen peroxide to water using a sulfhydryl (SH)-containing molecule, glutathione, as an electron donor. The glutathione-mediated reduction of hydrogen peroxide is written as follows:

$$H_2O_2 + 2\,GSH \rightarrow GSSG + 2\,H_2O \qquad (12.2)$$

where GSH is glutathione in the reduced state, and GSSG represents two oxidized glutathione molecules connected by a disul-

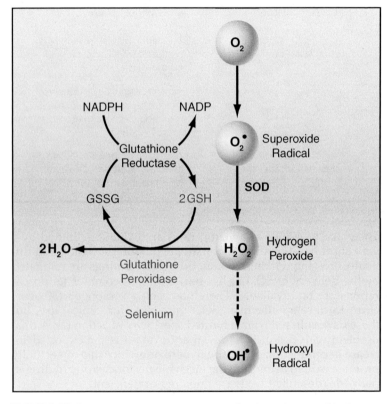

FIGURE 12.1 The glutathione redox system for the reduction of hydrogen peroxide to water. This system provides antioxidant protection by diverting hydrogen peroxide away from the production of hydroxyl radicals. See text for further explanation. GSH = the reduced form of glutathione, GSSG = the oxidized form of glutathione, SOD = superoxide dismutase.

fide bridge. The oxidized glutathione is then converted back to its reduced form by the enzyme, *glutathione reductase*, which uses NADPH as the electron donor. This series of reactions is shown in Figure 12.1.

Glutathione

As shown in Figure 12.2, glutathione is a tripeptide that contains glutamine, cysteine, and glycine moieties. The business portion of the molecule is a sulfhydryl (SH) group on cysteine, which allows glutathione to act as a reducing agent. (Molecules that contain SH groups are known as *thiols*.) Glutathione can also donate electrons to oxygen-derived free radicals, which is a method of antioxidant protection known as "scavenging."

Glutathione is the most abundant intracellular antioxidant in the body: it is synthesized in the cell cytoplasm and is maintained in millimolar concentrations in most cells. It must be in the reduced state (GSH) to act as an antioxidant, and the ratio of reduced to oxidized glutathione (GSH:GSSG) is normally about 100:1 (1). During periods of oxidative stress, this ratio can fall to 10:1, and even lower. Glutathione (hereafter abbreviated as GSH) can also move into extracellular fluid, but plasma levels are three orders of magnitude lower than intracellular levels. The most concentrated pool of extracellular GSH is in the epithelial lining fluid in the lungs, where the concentration is 140-fold higher than in plasma (8). This suggests that GSH is an important source of antioxidant protection in the lungs. In fact, GSH is an important antioxidant in all major organs of the human body (see later).

G6PD Deficiency

As indicated in Figure 12.1, the actions of NADPH serve to maintain intracellular GSH levels. The NADPH is generated by the pentose phosphate pathway, and one of the enzymes in this pathway is glucose-6-phosphate dehydrogenase (G6PD). Deficiency of the G6PD enzyme (a genetic defect that is present in over 400 million people worldwide) therefore results in GSH deficiency, which predisposes to oxidative cell injury. The principal consequence of this is hemolysis that is precipitated by oxidative stress (9).

Selenium

The glutathione peroxidase enzyme in humans requires the trace mineral selenium for its activity (10). The importance of selenium for antioxidant protection is suggested by a study of patients with severe sepsis and septic shock, where selenium levels in blood were abnormally low in all patients, and patients who received

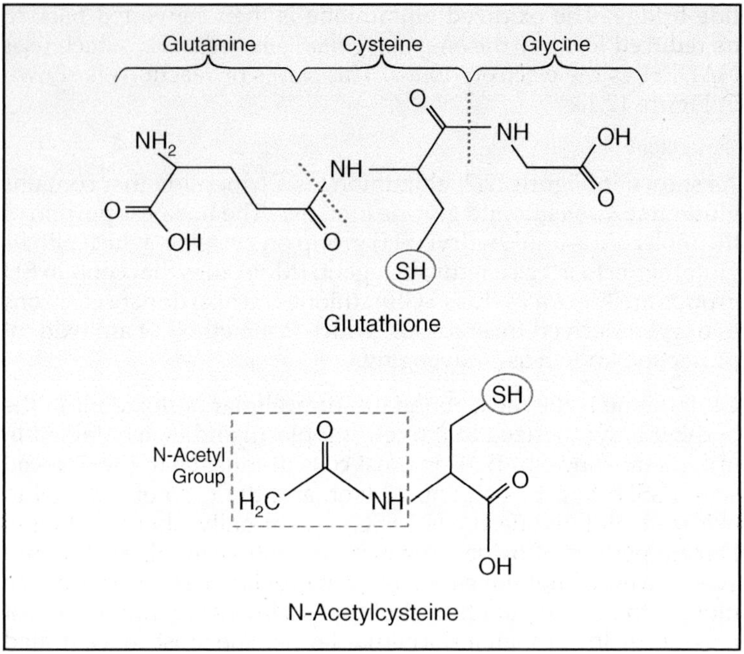

FIGURE 12.2 Structural formulas for glutathione (GSH) and N-acetylcysteine (NAC). The smaller NAC molecule can move into cells and provide the active ingredient (cysteine) for GSH production.

selenium infusions to raise the blood levels had a lower mortality rate (11).

Thiamine

Thiamine has an indirect role as an antioxidant because it serves as a cofactor for an enzyme in the pentose phosphate pathway that supplies the NADPH needed to keep GSH in its reduced form. Support for thiamine's role as an antioxidant is provided by animal studies showing that Wernicke's encephalopathy (induced by a thiamine-deficient diet) is accompanied by evidence of oxidative stress, and is partially corrected by thiamine administration (12).

Vitamin E

Vitamin E is a family of eight naturally occurring substances known as *tocols,* which are subdivided into four *tocopherols* and four *tocotrienols* (each designated as α, β, γ, and δ), with the latter class of molecules having more double bonds. The tocols are lipid soluble, and the predominant one in human tissues is α-*tocopherol*.

Antioxidant Actions

Cell membranes are rich in polyunsaturated fatty acids (PUFAs), which play an important role in maintaining the fluidity of cell membranes because of their low melting point. Unfortunately, PUFAs are highly oxidizable, and oxidized PUFAs polymerize and cause cell membranes to become stiff and leaky, which is a prelude to osmotic cell disruption. Vitamin E (α-tocopherol) protects membrane PUFAs from oxidation.

Because of its lipid solubility, α-tocopherol readily gains access to the lipid-rich interior of cell membranes, and what it does there is depicted in Figure 12.3. Shown is the reaction sequence for lipid peroxidation (shown in more detail in Figure 8.4), which is initiated by the action of a strong oxidant like the hydroxyl radical. This eventually leads to the production of a lipid peroxyl radical, which can oxidize a nearby PUFA and begin the reaction sequence anew. This creates a self-propagating "chain reaction." Alpha-tocopherol blocks this propagation, because lipid peroxyl radicals are about 1,000 times more likely to react with α-tocopherol than with PUFAs (13), and this reaction produces a relatively innocuous tocopheroxyl radical. Because of its ability to block the propagation of lipid peroxidation, α-tocopherol is often described as a "chain-breaking antioxidant."

Alpha-tocopherol is also found in lipoproteins, where it plays a similar role in blocking lipid peroxidation. The importance of this role is demonstrated by evidence that oxidation of both low-density and high-density lipoproteins (LDL and HDL, respectively) is instrumental in atherogenesis. (See page 131 for more on this topic.)

Vitamin C

Vitamin C (ascorbic acid) is a water-soluble vitamin that is best known for its essential role in collagen formation. However, it is also a reducing agent that can donate electrons to free radicals to erase their adverse effects. As a result, ascorbate can act as a "scavenger" for oxygen-derived free radicals: i.e., superoxide radicals, hydroxyl radicals, and peroxyl or alkoxyl radicals (14). Ascorbate also donates electrons to regenerate α-tocopherol (see Figure 12.3), although how this happens is not adequately

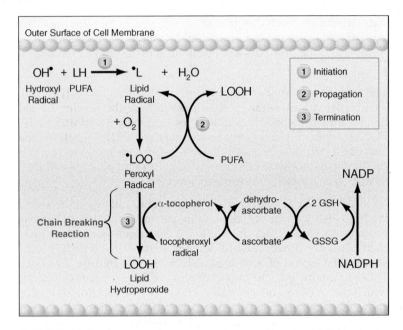

FIGURE 12.3 The antioxidant action of α-tocopherol, which blocks the propagation of lipid peroxidation. Note that vitamin C (ascorbate) and reduced glutathione (GSH) are involved in regenerating α-tocopherol. See text for further explanation. PUFA = polyunsaturated fatty acid.

explained, since ascorbate is water soluble, and α-tocopherol inhibits lipid-rich structures. The oxidized form of ascorbate (dehydroascorbate) is converted back to ascorbate with electrons donated by reduced glutathione (GSH).

Ascorbate is one of the most abundant antioxidants in extracellular fluids. It does not readily move into cells, as movement across cell membranes requires a specialized transporter, and low concentrations of ascorbate are typically found in cell cultures (14). There is evidence that ascorbate accumulates in activated neutrophils (15), presumably for protection against the explosion of reactive oxygen species produced during neutrophil activation.

Pro-Oxidant Effect?

Vitamin C increases iron absorption in the duodenum by donating electrons to convert ferric iron (Fe^{3+}) to ferrous iron (Fe^{2+}). This conversion also promotes the production of hydroxyl radicals from hydrogen peroxide (H_2O_2), as described by the following reaction:

$$H_2O_2 + Fe^{2+} \rightarrow Fe^{3+} + OH^{\cdot} + OH^{-} \qquad (12.3)$$

where $OH^{\cdot}$ is the hydroxyl radical, and OH^{-} is the hydroxyl ion. This is the well-known *Fenton reaction* (also described in Chapter 8), and the production of hydroxyl radicals from this reaction is a major source of oxidative cell injury. The ascorbate-initiated production of hydroxyl radicals has been repeatedly demonstrated *in vitro* (14), but the relevance of this pro-oxidant effect *in vivo* is uncertain. Of interest in this regard is a study showing that the combination of iron supplements (100 mg/day) and high-dose vitamin C (500 mg/day) produced evidence of lipid peroxidation in pregnant women who were not iron deficient (16). This suggests that high-dose vitamin C intake (i.e., >200 mg/day) carries a risk of pro-oxidant effects in subjects who are iron-overloaded.

An Epigenetic View

The ability to produce vitamin C is an ancestral trait in mammals, but has been lost in anthropoid primates (monkeys, apes, and us) as a result of a gene that no longer expresses the terminal enzyme in vitamin C synthesis (17). The gene is present but silent, suggesting an epigenetic change. Since the daily vitamin C intake is more than adequate in the affected species (18), it is possible that production of vitamin C was halted because it is not necessary. However, it is also possible that the gene silencing was a survival-promoting response to the pro-oxidant risk associated with vitamin C.

ANTIOXIDANT DEFICIENCY

The cessation of antioxidant production at the time of death is not the only instance where antioxidants fail us, because depletion of antioxidants often occurs during periods of severe or persistent oxidative stress.

Scope of The Problem

Depletion of endogenous antioxidants has been reported in a multitude of diseases, including those that are leading sources of morbidity and mortality. This is demonstrated in Table 12.2, which lists some of the prominent diseases that have been linked to glutathione (GSH) deficiency. The following are some relevant comments about the associations in this table.

TABLE 12.2 Conditions Associated with Glutathione Depletion

Category	Condition
Pulmonary Disorder	• ARDS (-80%)[†] • Severe COPD (-40%) • Cystic Fibrosis (-70%) • IPF (-80%)
ENT Disorders	• Rhinitis • Tonsillitis • Otitis media • Meniere Disease • Sclerosis of the Larynx and Tympanic Membranes
Neurogenerative Disorders	• ALS • Alzheimer Disease • Parkinson Disease
Hepatic Disorders	• Acetominophen Toxicity • Cirrhosis • Chronic Hepatitis C
Others	• AIDS • Cataracts • Mitochondrial Disorders • Sepsis/Septic Shock

[†]Numbers in parentheses indicate the percent decrease in GSH levels (µM) in the epithelial lining fluid in the lungs (20). ARDS = acute respiratory distress syndrome, IPF = idiopathic pulmonary fibrosis, ALS = amyotrophic lateral sclerosis.

Pulmonary Disorders

The lungs are exposed to higher concentrations of O_2 than any other internal organ in the body, so antioxidant protection is particularly important in the lungs. The relatively high concentration of GSH in the epithelial lining fluid of the lungs (i.e., 140 times higher than in plasma) (8) suggests that GSH plays an important role in protecting the lungs from oxidative injury. This is supported by animal studies showing that selective GSH deficiency increases the severity of pulmonary O_2 toxicity (19). Glutathione deficiency in the lungs has been reported in patients with severe COPD, cystic fibrosis, idiopathic pulmonary fibrosis, and the acute respiratory distress syndrome (ARDS), and Table 12.2 shows the severity of GSH depletion in each of these disorders (20,21).

ENT Disorders

The epithelial cells in the extrathoracic portion of the upper airway are exposed to atmospheric O_2 (or higher O_2 concentrations if supplemental O_2 is used), and also have a particularly high risk of oxidative damage. Glutathione is considered the principal antioxidant for these epithelial cells, and GSH deficiency has been documented in common inflammatory conditions in this region, including rhinitis (allergic and infectious), tonsillitis, and otitis media (22).

Neurodegenerative Disorders

Amyotrophic lateral sclerosis, Alzheimer's disease, and Parkinson's disease have all been linked to oxidative stress exacerbated by GSH depletion (23,24). Glutathione replacement therapy is hampered by the impermeability of the blood-brain barrier to GSH, but alternative forms of GSH delivery (e.g., liposomal formulations) are being evaluated (24).

Hepatic Disorders

In addition to its role as an antioxidant, GSH also participates in the elimination of drugs that are metabolized by the cytochrome P450 enzymes in the liver. This metabolic pathway produces reactive metabolites capable of oxidative cell injury. GSH forms conjugates with these metabolites, which has a detoxifying effect, and enhances drug elimination in the urine or feces. Excessive doses of a drug that is metabolized in this fashion can deplete GSH stores in the liver, and the subsequent buildup of the reactive metabolite promotes oxidative injury in the liver. This is the etiology of *acetaminophen hepatotoxicity*, which is the leading cause of acute liver failure in the United States, United Kingdom, Canada, Australia, and Scandinavia (25). The GSH replacement in this condition is provided by N-acetylcysteine, a precursor of GSH that is an effective antidote for acetaminophen overdoses (26). (More on N-acetylcysteine in the final section of the chapter.)

HIV Infection

Human immunodeficiency virus (HIV) infection is accompanied by reduced GSH levels in red blood cells and lymphocytes (including CD4 cells). This the result of cytokine-mediated inhibition of GSH synthesis, along with increased consumption of GSH in response to oxidative stress (27). Liposomal preparations of glutathione have been shown to restore the immune responses of CD4 cells to opportunistic infections (28), and this has fueled the hypothesis that oxidative stress is responsible for the altered viability of CD4 lymphocytes (and the subsequent propensity for opportunistic infections) in patients with HIV infection.

Sepsis/Septic Shock

Critically ill patients with persistent inflammation from sepsis or septic shock have the "perfect storm" for antioxidant deficiency; i.e., an increase in antioxidant consumption combined with inadequate intake. Therefore, it is no surprise that deficiencies of major antioxidants like GSH, vitamin C, and vitamin E are commonplace in these patients (29-32). Evidence that antioxidant deficiencies contribute to the organ dysfunction in septic shock is provided by *in vitro* studies using endothelial cells harvested from human umbilical veins. When these cells are exposed to plasma from patients with septic shock, there is a prompt increase in ROS production accompanied by a prompt decrease in intracellular GSH, and these changes precede an increase in the rate of cell death (33). This endothelial response is significantly muted if GSH or N-acetylcysteine is added prior to exposure to the septic plasma.

Septic shock is a leading cause of death in ICUs, and the mortality rate is directly related to the severity of oxidative stress (see Figure 9.4 in Chapter 9). This underscores the importance of antioxidant depletion in this condition.

Comment

A decrease in antioxidant levels can indicate that the antioxidant is being utilized to combat oxidative stress, which is not a detrimental condition. Absolute proof that a reduced antioxidant level is detrimental would require evidence that replenishing the antioxidant is accompanied by a decrease in oxidative stress. This is usually not possible because of problems with antioxidant delivery (see later). However, it is reasonable to assume that a diminished antioxidant level in the face of oxidative stress is evidence that antioxidant production is not matching the rate of utilization, which is a "red flag" for the possible exacerbation of oxidative stress.

Nutritional Considerations

Inadequate dietary intake is an underappreciated source of antioxidant deficiency. Although there is a Recommended Dietary Allowance (RDA) for many antioxidants, the RDA reflects the minimum requirements in healthy subjects and may underestimate what is needed during periods of oxidative stress. Reduced dietary intake is common in acutely ill or seriously ill patients, and in the elderly.

Glutathione

Glutathione (GSH) is synthesized *de novo* in cells, but its three component amino acids (glutamine, cysteine, and glycine) are "conditionally essential," which means that dietary sources are needed during periods of increased metabolic activity. In addition, since the antioxidant actions of GSH are the result of a sulfhydryl (SH) group on the cysteine moiety, a dietary source of sulfur is needed to maintain cysteine production. (This dietary source is provided by another sulfur-containing amino acid, methionine.) There is a rapid turnover of GSH in all tissues (e.g., the half-life of GSH is <1 hour in the kidneys) (34), so a steady supply of sulfur is needed to maintain GSH production.

The rapid turnover of GSH is reflected in a study of fasting in healthy adults, where there was a significant decrease in intracellular GSH levels after four days, and by the seventh day, GSH levels had dropped by 50% (see Figure 13.3) (35). Similar results have been observed in animal studies, where a three-day fast has produced a 41% decrease in GSH levels in the lungs (36). More severe changes are expected in the presence of oxidative stress.

ANTIOXIDANT THERAPY

Despite the reports of antioxidant depletion in a multitude of diseases involving oxidative stress, the cumulative experience with antioxidant replacement therapy has not matched expectations. Clinical trials of antioxidant therapy have produced either negative or inconsistent results. However, the problems seem to be methodological rather than conceptual, and some of these problems are briefly described here.

Drug Delivery

A major problem with the administration of endogenous antioxidants is *limited bioavailability* (i.e., the extent to which an administered drug reaches the desired site of action.) This has been demonstrated for all of the endogenous antioxidants, but especially for the antioxidant enzymes (which do not pass through cell membranes) and GSH (which has a short half-life in plasma, and does not readily pass into cells). The following are some available measures for improving the bioavailability of antioxidants.

N-Acetylcysteine

N-acetylcysteine (NAC) is an acetylated derivative of the amino acid cysteine that is essentially the business portion of the GSH molecule (see Figure 12.2). It was first introduced as a mucolytic agent (Mucomyst™) because of its ability to break disulfide bonds between mucoproteins in sputum (37). In the 1980s, NAC emerged as an effective antidote for acetaminophen hepatotoxicity (26), which (as described earlier) is a result of GSH depletion in the liver. This demonstrated that NAC could cross cell membranes and supplement intracellular GSH levels.

The discovery that NAC can promote intracellular GSH levels led to an investigation of NAC in pulmonary O_2 toxicity, and the results are shown in Figure 12.4 (38). The inhalation of 100% O_2 for 7 days (in laboratory mice) resulted in a 47% decrease in GSH levels in the lungs and a 78% mortality rate, and the administration of NAC dropped the mortality rate to 28%. Since the time of this study (in 1985), NAC has been evaluated as an antioxidant in a wide variety of conditions involving every major organ in the body. (A recent review includes studies of NAC in about 50 different diseases.) (39). The results of these evaluations are mixed (39,40), but the number of favorable results seems to match, or even exceed, the unfavorable ones. One of the shortcomings of the available studies of NAC is the dosing, which is usually far below the dosage used to promote GSH production in acetaminophen overdoses. NAC has a favorable safety profile, and more aggressive dosing is warranted. Overall, NAC is a promising antioxidant and deserves continued study.

Liposomes

Drug delivery to tissue sites can be facilitated by encasing the drugs in liposomes, which are spherical vesicles composed of a phospholipid bilayer surrounding an aqueous core. These "nanovehicles" can transport both lipid-soluble and water-soluble drugs, and a coating of polyethylene glycol prevents immune recognition. Liposomes can also be equipped with tissue-specific ligands for more targeted drug delivery.

Liposomes have improved antioxidant delivery and efficacy in both *in vitro* studies (41) and animal studies (42). However, there are no clinical studies of liposomal antioxidant therapy to date. The reason for this is unclear, but liposomal drug delivery is a costly endeavor, and it is possible that liposomal antioxidant therapy is in a "Catch 22" conundrum (where some success in antioxidant therapy is needed to justify the cost and effort of liposomal therapy, but liposomal therapy is needed to produce some success in antioxidant therapy). Whatever the reason, liposomes have been available for targeted drug delivery for over 50 years, and it seems unlikely that they will be used for antioxidant therapy in the near (or distant) future.

Other Problems

Some additional problems with studies of antioxidant therapy are summarized below.

1. The primary end point of many studies is a global outcome measure, like mortality rate, that can have a multitude of determining factors. The efficacy of antioxidant therapy should be evaluated by a measure of oxidative stress.

2. In many of the long-term studies of antioxidant therapy (e.g., for heart disease), antioxidants are given without evidence of deficiency. This is problematic, because many antioxidants

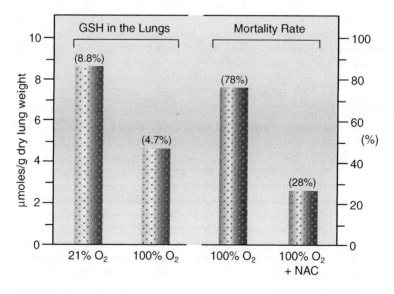

FIGURE 12.4 The effect of hyperoxia on glutathione (GSH) levels in the lungs (left panel), and the effect of GSH replacement with N-acetylcysteine (NAC) on the mortality from hyperoxic lung injury (right panel). Data from Reference 38.

(e.g., ascorbic acid) are promptly excreted and lost if there is not an underlying deficiency.

3. Most studies use a fixed dosage of antioxidants, but the appropriate dosing regimens for antioxidants is unknown, and several dosing levels should be evaluated.

4. Studies on antioxidant therapy characteristically focus on an individual chemical species. However, oxidative stress may be a multifaceted condition, and replacing one antioxidant will not resolve the problem if there are deficiencies in other antioxidants. Therefore, a more complex approach to antioxidant therapy, which includes monitoring a host of antioxidants, seems warranted.

Comment

The lack of a consistent benefit with antioxidant therapy is often interpreted as evidence against the importance of oxidative stress. However, taking direction from the introductory quote by Carl Sagan, *the lack of an expected response to antioxidant therapy does not dismiss the existence of oxidative tissue injury*. Instead, it indicates an inadequacy in the treatment regimen. This is no different than the all-too-frequent episodes of treatments we prescribe that do not have the desired effect. Failed treatments do not negate the diseases we are trying to treat.

SUMMATION

The human body is equipped with a robust system of antioxidant protection that helps to keep oxidation at bay during our lifetime. This chapter describes the workings of this system, using the most studied of our endogenous antioxidants. Some of the relevant points in the chapter are as follows.

1. A major mechanism of antioxidant protection is the reduction of hydrogen peroxide directly to water, which circumvents the production of highly destructive hydroxyl radicals. The principal enzyme for this reaction is glutathione peroxidase, which engineers the transfer of electrons from glutathione to hydrogen peroxide. This enzyme requires selenium as a cofactor (in humans).

2. Glutathione is a tripeptide that acts as an antioxidant by virtue of a sulfhydryl (SH) group on one of its amino acids (cysteine). It is present in abundance in all cells, and is considered the major intracellular antioxidant in the body. It must

be kept in the reduced state (GSH) to donate electrons and thereby function as an antioxidant.

3. A member of the vitamin E family, α-tocopherol, is a major lipid-soluble antioxidant that blocks lipid peroxidation in cell membranes and circulating lipoproteins.

4. Vitamin C (ascorbic acid) is a major water-soluble antioxidant that inactivates (scavenges) reactive oxygen species and keeps α-tocopherol in its active (reduced) form.

5. In conditions where oxidative stress plays a role, antioxidant depletion is a common and often unrecognized contributing factor.

6. Studies evaluating the therapeutic potential of endogenous antioxidants have been hampered by the limitations in bioavailability. N-acetylcysteine overcomes the limited bioavailability of GSH because it readily enters cells and serves as a precursor for GSH production.

REFERENCES

a. Sagan C. The Demon Haunted World; Science as a Candle in the Dark. New York: Random House Publishing Group, 1996.

1. Halliwell B, Gutteridge JMC. Antioxidant defenses synthesized in vivo. In: Free Radicals in Biology and Medicine. 5th ed. Oxford: Oxford University Press, 2015: 77-152.

2. McCord JM, Fridovich I. Superoxide dismutase. An enzymatic function for erythrocuprein (hemocuprein). J Biol Chem 1969; 244:6049-6055.

3. Lane N. Oxygen: The Molecule That Made the World. Oxford: Oxford University Press, 2002.

4. Lebovitz RM, Khang H, Vogel H, et al. Neurodegeneration, myocardial injury, and perinatal death in mitochondrial superoxide dismutase-deficient mice. Proc Natl Acad Sci 1996; 93:9782-9787.

5. White CW, Avraham KB, Shanley PF, Groner Y. Transgenic mice with expression of elevated levels of copper-zinc superoxide dismutase in the lungs are resistant to pulmonary oxygen toxicity. J Clin Invest 1991; 87:2162-2168.

6. Turrena JF, Crapo JD, Freeman BA. Protection against oxygen toxicity by intravenous injection of liposome-entrapped catalase and superoxide dismutase. J Clin Invest 1984; 73:87-95.

7. Batinic-Haberle I, Tome ME. Thiol regulation by Mn porphyrins, commonly known as SOD mimetics. Redox Biol 2019; 25:101139.

8. Cantin AM, North SL, Hubbard RC, Crystal RG. Normal epithelial lining fluid contains high levels of glutathione. J Appl Physiol 1987; 63:152-157.

9. Capellini MD, Fiorelli G. Glucose-6-phosphate dehydrogenase defi-

ciency. Lancet 2008; 371:64-74.

10. Lubos E, Loscalzo J, Handy DE. Glutathione peroxidase-1 in health and disease: from molecular mechanisms to therapeutic opportunities. Antiox Redox Signal 2011; 15:1957-1997.

11. Selenium in Intensive Care (SIC): results of a prospective randomized, placebo-controlled, multiple-center study in patients with severe systemic inflammatory response syndrome, sepsis, and septic shock. Crit Care Med 2007; 35:118-126.

12. Zarros A, Liapi C, Al-Humadi H, et al. Experimentally-induced Wernicke's encephalopathy modifies crucial rat brain parameters: the importance of Na^+, K^+-ATPase and a potentially neuroprotective role for antioxidant supplementation. Met Brain Res 2013; 28:387-396.

13. Halliwell B, Gutteridge JMC. Antioxidants from the diet. In: Free Radicals in Biology and Medicine. 5th ed. Oxford: Oxford University Press, 2015: 153-198.

14. Smirnoff N. Ascorbic acid metabolism and functions: A comparison of plants and mammals. Free Radic Biol Med 2018; 122:116-129.

15. Wang Y, Russo TA, Kwon O, et al. Ascorbate recycling in human neutrophils: Induction by bacteria. Proc Natl Acad Sci 1997; 94:13816-13819.

16. Lachili B, Hininger I, Faure H, et al. Increased lipid peroxidation in pregnant women after iron and vitamin C supplementation. Biol Trace Elem Res 2001; 83:103-110.

17. Drouin G, Godin J-R, Pagé, B. The genetics of vitamin C loss in vertebrates. Curr Genom 2011; 12:371-378.

18. Food and Nutrition Board, Institute of Medicine. Dietary Reference Intakes for Vitamin C, vitamin E, selenium, and carotenoids. Washington, DC: National Academy Press, 2000.

19. Deneke SM, Lynch BA, Sanberg BL. Transient depletion of lung glutathione by diethylmaleate enhances oxygen toxicity. J Appl Physiol 1985; 58:571-574.

20. Gould NS, Day BJ. Targeting maladaptive glutathione responses in lung disease. Biochem Pharmacol 2011; 81:187-193.

21. Pacht ER, Timerman AP, Lykens MG, Merola AJ. Deficiency of alveolar fluid glutathione in patients with sepsis and the adult respiratory distress syndrome. Chest 1991; 100:1397-1403.

22. Asher BF, Guilford FT. Oxidative stress and low glutathione in common ear, nose, and throat conditions: a systematic review. Altern Ther Health Med 2016; 22:44-50.

23. Gu F, Chauhan V, Chauhan A. Glutathione redox imbalance in brain disorders. Curr Opin Clin Nutr Metab Care 2015; 18:89-95.

24. Cacciatore I, Baldassarre L, Fornasari E. et al. Recent advances in the treatment of neurodegenerative diseases based on GSH delivery systems. Oxid Med Cell Longev 2012; 2012:240146.

25. Kalsi SS, Dargan PI, Waring WS, Wood DM. A review of the evidence

concerning hepatic glutathione depletion and susceptibility to hepatotoxicity after paracetamol overdose. Open Access Emerg Med 2011; 3:87-96.

26. Buckley NA, Whyte IM, O'Connell DL, et al. Oral or intravenous N-acetylcysteine: which is the treatment of choice for acetaminophen (paracetamol) poisoning? J Toxicol Clin Toxicol 1999; 37:759-767.

27. Morris D, Guerra C, Donohue C, et al. Unveiling the mechanisms for decreased glutathione in individuals with HIV infection. Clin Dev Immunol 2012; 2012:734125.

28. Ly J, Lagman M, Saing T, et al. Liposomal glutathione supplementation restores TH1 cytokine response to Mycobacterium tuberculosis infection in HIV-infected animals. J Interferon Cytokine Res 2015; 35:875-887.

29. Fläring UB, Rooyackers OE, Hebert C, et al. Temporal changes in whole-blood and plasma glutathione in ICU patients with multiple organ failure. Intensive Care Med 2005; 31:1072-1078.

30. Pincemail J, Bertrans Y, Hanique G, et al. Evaluation of vitamin E deficiency in patients with adult respiratory distress syndrome. Ann NY Acad Sci 1989; 570:498-500.

31. Fain O, Pariés J, Jacquart B, et al. Hypovitaminosis C in hospitalized patients. Eur J Intern Med 2003; 14:419-425.

32. Marik P, Khangoora V, Rivera R, et al. Hydrocortisone, vitamin C, and thiamine for the treatment of severe sepsis and septic shock. Chest 2017; 151:1229-1238.

33. Huet O, Cherreau C, Nicco C, et al. Pivotal role of glutathione depletion in plasma-induced endothelial oxidative stress during sepsis. Crit Care Med 2008; 36:2328-2334.

34. Kosower NS, Kosower EM. The glutathione status of cells. Int Rev Cytol 1978; 54:109-160.

35. Martensson J The effect of fasting on leukocyte and plasma glutathione and sulfur amino acid concentrations. Metab 1986; 35:118-121.

36. Smith LJ, Anderson J, Shamsuddin M, Hsueh W. Effect of fasting on hyperoxic lung injury in mice. Role of glutathione. Am Rev Respir Dis 1990; 141:141-149.

37. Aldini G, Altomere A, Baron G, et al. N-Acetylcysteine as an antioxidant and disulfide breaking agent: the reasons why. Free Rad Res 2018; 52:751-762.

38. Patterson CE, Butler JA, Byrne JA, Rhodes ML. Oxidant lung injury: intervention with sulfhydryl agents. Lung 1985; 163:23-32.

39. Schwalfenberg GK. N-Acetylcysteine: a review of clinical usefulness (an old drug with new tricks). J Nutr Metab 2021; 2021:9949453.

40. Tenório MCdS, Graciliano NG, Moura FA, et al. N-Acetylcysteine (NAC) Impacts on human health. Antiox 2021; 10:967.

41. Zeevalk GD, Bernard LP, and Guilford FT. Liposomal-glutathione provides maintenance of intracellular glutathione and neuroprotection in mesencephalic neuronal cells. Neurochem Res 2010; 35:1575-1587.

When is oxygen therapy safe?

13

> "In the final analysis, if we could safely and effectively protect against oxygen toxicity, we could use oxygen therapy with impunity…"
>
> Barry Fanburg (1)

The question in the title of this chapter was addressed in an editorial published in 1988 that concerned oxygen toxicity in critically ill patients (1). This editorial (written by a prominent pulmonary and critical care specialist) emphasized the role of endogenous antioxidants in protecting against oxygen toxicity, and recommended vigilance for antioxidant depletion in patients at risk of pulmonary oxygen toxicity (e.g., ventilator-dependent patients and those with high oxygen requirements). This attention to antioxidant protection is reflected in one of the concluding remarks in the editorial, which is the introductory quote for this chapter.

Flash forward 33 years (to 2021), and the standard practice for preventing pulmonary O_2 toxicity is to limit the concentration of inhaled O_2, with no regard for the status of antioxidant protection in the lungs. This chapter will demonstrate the folly of this practice, beginning with a brief history of how oxygen, and its toxic manifestations, were discovered.

HISTORICAL BACKGROUND

The Greek philosopher Empedocles was the first to propose (circa 450 B.C.) that all matter is represented by four indivisible elements: earth, air, fire, and water. This became the accepted dogma for over 2,000 years, but it did not survive the second half of the 18th century, thanks to the discovery of oxygen. The following is a brief account of the men responsible for the discovery of oxygen, and its inherent toxicity.

Joseph Priestley

Joseph Priestley was an 18th century English theologian and dissident who was actively involved in the field of "pneumatic chemistry" (the study of gases or "airs"). On August 1, 1774, Priestley produced a gas by heating a sample of mercuric oxide (HgO) and noted that "a candle burned in this air with a remarkable vigorous flame" (2). He had triggered the following reaction:

$$2\,HgO + heat \rightarrow 2\,Hg + O_2 \qquad (13.1)$$

The gas was pure oxygen, but Priestley erroneously interpreted the result because of his belief in the *phlogiston theory of combustion*, which claimed that substances burn because they contain a fire-promoting element called phlogiston, which is released into the air during the burning process. When the air is saturated with phlogiston, the burning ceases. Priestley thus concluded that the flame-enhancing gas was devoid of phlogiston (which would facilitate the release of phlogiston from the burning material), and he named the gas "dephlogisticated air."

Priestley had one concern with the flame-enhancing, dephlogisticated gas, which he stated as follows (2):

> … for, as a candle burns out much faster in dephlogisticated than in common air, so we might, as may be said, *live out too fast*, and the animal powers be too soon exhausted, in this pure kind of air.

Thus, although Joseph Priestley erred in identifying his flame-enhancing gas, he was "spot on" in identifying the destructive potential of the gas.

(*Note:* Three years before Priestley's experiment, a Swedish chemist named Carl Wilhelm Scheele produced oxygen by heating mercuric oxide. He called the gas "fire-air" but, like Priestley, he interpreted his findings according to the phlogiston theory of combustion. Scheele did not publish his findings for several years; as a result, he has been relegated to the background in historical accounts of how oxygen was discovered.)

Antoine Lavoisier

Shortly after Priestley produced the flame-enhancing gas, he traveled to France on vacation and had the opportunity to describe his findings to the celebrated French chemist, Antoine Lavoisier. Lavoisier had been skeptical of the phlogiston theory because he had noted that metals gain in weight when they burn, yet they should lose weight if burning releases phlogiston. He also had a dim view of Joseph Priestley, whose work he regarded as "a fabric of experiments hardly interrupted by any reasoning"(3). Nevertheless, Lavoisier repeated Priestley's experiment and produced the flame-enhancing gas. He then heated a sample of mercury that was placed in the gas, using an apparatus like the one in Figure 13.1. (Lavoisier was reversing the chemical process that produced the gas.) The mercury gained weight while burning, and the gas lost an equivalent amount of weight, so Lavoisier concluded that the fire-promoting element was in the gas, not in the burning material. He named this element "oxygene"(4), which means "acid producer" (based on Lavoisier's misconception that reactions with oxygen always generate acids).

Thus did Lavoisier simultaneously debunk the 100-year dominance of the phlogiston theory of combustion, and the 2,000-year belief that air was a single, indivisible element. Lavoisier presented his findings in 1777, but he neglected to mention Priestley's contribution; as a result, he was credited with the discovery of oxygen. In the many years he worked with oxygen, Lavoisier reported no adverse effects, although he did notice that the laboratory mice looked sickly when left in a pure O_2 environment for more than a few hours (3).

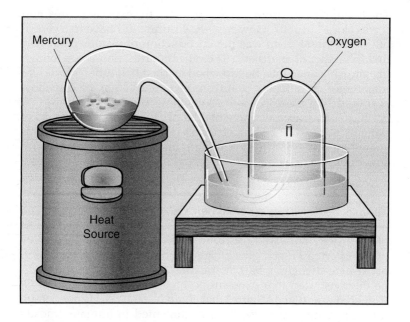

FIGURE 13.1 The apparatus used by Antoine Lavoisier in the discovery of oxygen. See text for explanation.

Thomas Beddoes

Based on Lavoisier's work with oxygen, an enterprising British physician named Thomas Beddoes opened the first Pneumatic Institute (in 1798), where the inhalation of O_2 and other "factitious gases" would be used to treat a variety of diseases, especially tuberculosis (which was responsible for one of every four deaths in England at the time). Beddoes was aware of Lavoisier's observations on the sickly behavior of animals after prolonged exposure to 100% O_2, so he conducted an experiment (using kittens) where one animal was exposed to 80% O_2 for 17 hours, and another was left breathing room air (5). The animals were then euthanized, and the one exposed to high O_2 was noted to have inflammation in the lungs and pleura, which was not present in the control animal. Beddoes concluded (5):

> It appears that oxygene air, when inspired pure, or nearly so, increases the internal motions for as to produce dangerous and mortal inflammation.

This is probably the first documented report of tissue injury from hyperoxia.

The Pneumatic Institute failed to produce the expected cures, and it was closed in 1807. However, the Institute did have two contributions. One of them was the introduction of nitrous oxide, the first inhalational anesthetic. The other contribution is the following amusing anecdote. Beddoes had learned that tuberculosis was uncommon in butchers, and from this observation, he somehow surmised that there could be something in a cow's breath that eradicates the disease. Therefore, he placed cows in the rooms of patients with advanced tuberculosis (6), only to discover that his "cow-house therapy" did nothing more than fill the rooms with cow dung.

Paul Bert

Thomas Beddoes' report on hyperoxia and inflammation sparked little interest, and almost 100 years passed before the next report of O_2 toxicity appeared (in 1878). This came from the laboratory of Paul Bert, a French physiologist who was studying the effects of extreme changes in barometric pressure. Using dogs and birds, he demonstrated that exposure to ≥5 atmospheres (ATM) of O_2 triggered grand mal seizures that could be fatal (7). Hyperoxia-induced seizures have also been documented in humans (mostly from studies in underwater divers), and a seizure threshold of 1.7 ATM (of 100% O_2) has been identified (8). (This corresponds to a PO_2 of 1,292 mm Hg at sea level.) However, there is a large variability in seizure threshold, and tolerance to 3 ATMs (PO_2 = 2,280 mm Hg at sea level) has been documented in individual test subjects (8).

James Lorrain Smith

About 20 years after Paul Bert's discovery of central nervous system O_2 toxicity, a Scottish pathologist named James Lorrain Smith studied less severe degrees of hyperoxia, and noted that laboratory mice exposed to 100% O_2 at 0.74 – 0.8 ATM developed respiratory failure without seizure activity, and died after an average of 4 days (9). The following is Lorrain Smith's description of the microscopic findings in the lungs of mice that inhaled 100% O_2 at 1.3 ATM for 90 hours (9):

> The alveoli were to a great extent filled with an exudate, which was granular and fibrillated … There were no microorganisms to be found. This pneumonic condition was universal …

This picture of diffuse exudative pulmonary edema is the first description of the microsopic changes in pulmonary oxygen toxicity.

NORMOBARIC OXYGEN TOXICITY

Prolonged breathing of O_2 at a pressure of 1 ATM produces a diffuse inflammatory injury in the lungs that is very similar to the pathological changes in the *acute respiratory distress syndrome* (ARDS). The process begins with oxidative damage in the endothelial lining of the pulmonary capillaries (10,11). This promotes the adhesion, and activation, of circulating neutrophils, and the associated increase in capillary permeability leads to the invasion of the pulmonary parenchyma by an inflammatory exudate. Oxidative changes in lung macrophages leads to the release of proinflammatory cytokines, which perpetuates the inflammatory invasion of the lungs. Persistent inflammation then leads to irreversible fibrosis and pulmonary hypertension (11). Alveolar epithelial cells are resistant to hyperoxic injury in many, but not all, of the animal species studied (10,11).

Variability

Most of the experimental studies on pulmonary O_2 toxicity have been performed on animals, and there is a significant variability in the susceptibility to O_2 toxicity in different species. This is shown in Table 13.1 (12-14). Some of the differences (i.e., between

TABLE 13.1   Interspecies Variability in the Risk of Oxygen Toxicity

Species	Survival with 100% O_2
Cold-Blooded Animals Frogs Sea Turtles	Several Weeks
Fowl Chickens Quail	10 - 15 days
Nonhuman Primates Baboons Monkeys	4 - 7 days
Small Animals Guinea Pigs Hamsters Mice Rats	2 - 5 days
Humans	??

From References 12-14.

cold-blooded animals and small animals) may be explained by the metabolic rate, which has a direct relationship with the risk of oxidative injury. There is also a variability within species based on gender (i.e., males have a higher risk than females) and age (i.e., adult animals have a higher risk than immature animals) (11).

Human Studies

Conducting experiments to identify the lethal dose of O_2 is not feasible in humans, but healthy volunteers have been exposed to 100% O_2 for up to 48 hours (15). The earliest sign of O_2 toxicity is a tracheobronchitis that produces a dry cough and chest pain. The onset is from 4 to 22 hours (11), and it precedes any changes in pulmonary function. The earliest evidence of pulmonary parenchymal involvement is a decrease in vital capacity, which is reported at 25-30 hours (15). However, vital capacity is not a sensitive marker of tissue events, since bronchoalveolar lavage after 17 hours of breathing >95% O_2 has shown an increased albumin concentration in the lavage fluid, indicating an alveolar-capillary leak (16). Exposure to 100% O_2 for only 2 hours has resulted in evidence of lipid peroxidation in the lungs, as determined by an increase in pentane (a volatile product of lipid peroxidation) in exhaled breath (17).

Patients who require high concentrations of inhaled O_2 typically have severe cardiopulmonary dysfunction, and many require mechanical ventilation. The influence of lung disease on the susceptibility to O_2 toxicity is unknown, but there is evidence that *hyperoxia is more damaging when combined with mechanical ventilation* (18). There is one human study that evaluated prolonged (60-70 hours) exposure to 100% O_2 during mechanical ventilation (19). This study involved 10 patients who met brain death criteria and had no cardiopulmonary disease: 5 patients were ventilated on room air, and 5 patients received 100% O_2. Mechanical ventilation was continued for over 60 hours. The patients exposed to hyperoxia developed a significant decrement in alveolar-capillary O_2 exchange after 40 hours, but there were no other differences from the patients ventilated on room air (including microscopic examination of postmortem lung specimens).

The limited experience with prolonged hyperoxia in humans makes it difficult to determine the susceptibility to hyperoxic lung injury. Further complicating the issue, there are several factors that influence the risk of hyperoxic lung injury, independent of species. These factors are listed in Table 13.2. Note the protective effect of low-level O_2 breathing for 3 – 5 days (presumably from induced production of antioxidants) (11). The factor at the top of the list in Table 13.2 is the focus of the next section.

ANTIOXIDANT DEPLETION

The greatest risk of hyperoxic lung injury occurs in critically ill patients, who are often ventilator dependent, malnourished, hypermetabolic, and receiving relatively high concentrations of inhaled oxygen. Unfortunately, antioxidant depletion is commonplace in these patients (20-23), as described in Chapter 12. The aggravating effect of antioxidant depletion on pulmonary O_2 toxicity is demonstrated in Figure 13.2 (24).

TABLE 13.2	Factors that Influence the Risk of Hyperoxic Lung Injury
Increased Risk	1. Antioxidant depletion (e.g., from malnutrition) 2. HIV infection (via selective glutathione depletion) 3. Mechanical ventilation (especially with high tidal volumes) 4. Increased metabolic rate (e.g., from epinephrine, sepsis, fever) 5. Pulmonary diseases that promote oxidative stress (?) 6. Advanced age 7. Chemotherapeutic agents (e.g., bleomycin, methotrexate) 8. Ongoing radiotherapy
Decreased Risk	1. Low-level O_2 breathing for 3-5 days 2. Decreased metabolic rate (e.g. hypothermia)

The source of antioxidant depletion in critically ill patients is an increase in utilization (typically in response to inflammatory diseases that increase production of reactive oxygen species) combined with an inadequate dietary intake. There is also evidence that pulmonary O_2 toxicity depletes antioxidants (see Figure 12.4 in Chapter 12) (25), which creates a positive feedback loop that can lead to rapid progression of hyperoxic lung injury.

Dietary Intake

Nutritional support in ventilator-dependent patients is usually provided by liquid feeding formulas delivered into the stomach or duodenum. Feeding regimens provide the Recommended Dietary Allowance (RDA) for nutrients that promote antioxidant protection, like zinc, copper, manganese, selenium, vitamins A, C, and E, plus amino acids. However, the RDA reflects the minimum requirements for the preservation of health (not for the return to health), and it likely underestimates what is needed during periods of oxidative stress. In addition, nutrient intake can be reduced from episodes where tube feedings are held because of regurgitation or high gastric residual volumes.

Glutathione

Glutathione (GSH) is a sulfhydryl-containing tripeptide (glutamine, cysteine, and glycine) that is a major intracellular antioxidant, and a major source of antioxidant protection in the lungs (see Chapter 12). This antioxidant is often overlooked in dietary considerations because it is produced *de novo* in cells. However, the diet remains an important determinant of intracellular GSH for the following reasons. First, the amino acid components of GSH are "conditionally essential," which means that dietary sources are needed during periods of increased metabolic activity. Second, the antioxidant actions of GSH are the result of a sulfhydryl (SH) group on the cysteine moiety, so a dietary source of sulfur is needed to maintain cysteine production. (The sulfur-containing amino acid, methionine, is a typical source of dietary sulfur.) Finally, there is a rapid turnover of GSH (e.g., the half-life of GSH is less than one hour in the kidneys) (26), so a steady supply of sulfur is needed to maintain GSH production.

The importance of dietary intake for maintaining GSH levels is shown in Figure 13.3. In this case, healthy adults were placed on a seven-day fast, and GSH levels in circulating leukocytes were

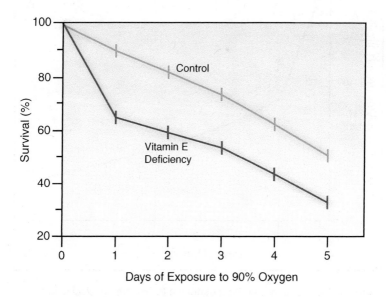

FIGURE 13.2 Effect of vitamin E deficiency (produced by dietary restriction) on the mortality rate in laboratory rats breathing 90% oxygen. Data from Reference 24.

monitored (27). Note the steady decline in intracellular GSH, which reaches a 50% reduction from baseline after 7 days. Similar results have been observed in animal studies, where a three-day fast resulted in a 41% decrease in GSH levels in the lungs (28). A more drastic decline in GSH levels is expected in the presence of oxidative stress.

Comment

The conventional practice has been to define the risk of hyperoxic lung injury solely in terms of the fractional concentration of inspired O_2 (FIO_2). The popular answer to the question in the title of this chapter would be that O_2 therapy is safe for all patients when the FIO_2 is $\leq 50\%$. This number is based on studies showing that higher FIO_2 levels are accompanied by an increase in venous

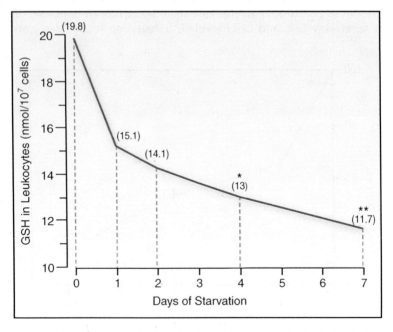

FIGURE 13.3 Changes in the glutathione (GSH) level in circulating leukocytes during a seven-day fast in eight healthy adults. Numbers in parentheses represent mean values. The asterisk indicates a significant change ($p<0.05$) from baseline (at zero hours), and the double asterisk indicates a significant change ($p<0.05$) from the prior measurement. Data from Reference 27.

admixture (a manifestation of intrapulmonary shunting) (29). However, this is an acute hemodynamic effect of oxygen (i.e., pulmonary vasodilation with an increase in pulmonary blood flow), which has no relationship to pulmonary O_2 toxicity; a condition characterized by inflammatory lung injury.

Considering the uncertainty about the susceptibility to hyperoxic lung injury in humans, and the multiple factors that influence this susceptibility (in Table 13.2), the appropriate answer to the question in the title of this chapter would be that *it is not possible to identify a level of inspired oxygen that is safe or toxic in any individual patient*. Information about the status of antioxidant protection (and the other factors in Table 13.2) is critical for assessing the risk of pulmonary O_2 toxicity.

Antioxidant Status

The current practice of ignoring antioxidant depletion will underestimate the risk of hyperoxic lung injury; as a result, hyperoxic lung injury is probably more common than suspected in patients who are seriously ill, ventilator dependent, or malnourished (since antioxidant depletion is commonplace in these patients). Monitoring the status of antioxidants, like GSH, vitamin C, vitamin E, and selenium, should be adopted for these patients, along with attempts to correct any deficiencies.

Exhaled Breath Analysis

The risk of hyperoxic lung injury is best evaluated by a measure of oxidative stress in the lungs. This measure is possible, because lipid peroxidation generates volatile byproducts that can be measured in the exhaled breath. There are several volatile byproducts, including alkanes (pentane, ethane, and octane) and aldehydes (pentanal and hexanal). Each has been measured in exhaled breath condensates, and elevated levels have been used as markers of inflammation and oxidative injury in the lungs (17,30). Unfortunately, exhaled breath analysis is not available for patient care. (There is a company in the Netherlands called eNose that has a device for exhaled breath analysis, but their current focus is lung cancer and colon cancer.)

SUMMATION

The focus of this chapter is "normobaric" O_2 toxicity and the factors that enhance or diminish the susceptibility to O_2 toxicity. The aim is to debunk the current dogma about the risk of hyperoxic lung injury. The following points are relevant:

1. Most of the current knowledge about pulmonary O_2 toxicity comes from animal studies, especially small animals like laboratory mice and rats. However, the susceptibility to O_2 toxicity varies in different species, and it is highest in the animals that are most often studied: small laboratory animals. Therefore, much of the data on pulmonary O_2 toxicity cannot be applied to humans.

2. The risk of hyperoxic lung injury is increased by mechanical ventilation and antioxidant depletion, and both conditions are common in critically ill patients.

3. The standard teaching that an FIO_2 >50% represents a risk for hyperoxic lung injury is based on the observed increase in intrapulmonary shunting that occurs at an FIO_2 above 50%. However, this is the result of an oxygen-induced ventilation-perfusion mismatch, which is unrelated to the inflammatory lung injury that characterizes pulmonary O_2 toxicity.

4. There is no regard for the status of antioxidant protection when assessing the risk of hyperoxic lung injury, and this is problematic in seriously ill patients because antioxidant depletion is commonplace in these patients. As a result, the risk of hyperoxic lung injury is underestimated, and the condition is more common than suspected.

5. Monitoring the status of antioxidant protection should be an adopted practice during oxygen therapy for patients who are ventilator dependent, malnourished, or breathing hyperoxic gas mixtures.

6. Ultimately, the risk of hyperoxic lung injury should be assessed using a measure of oxidant stress in the lungs. Expiratory gas analysis may provide that measure, but it is not currently available for patient care.

REFERENCES

1. Fanburg BL. Oxygen toxicity: why can't a human be more like a turtle. J Intensive Care Med 1988; 3:134-136.

2. Priestley J. Experiments and observations on different kinds of air. London: J. Johnson, 1775. In: Fulton JF, Wilson LG, eds. Selected Readings in the History of Physiology. 2nd ed., Springfield: Charles C Thomas, 1966:127-132.

3. Bell MS. Lavoisier in the Year One: The Birth of a New Science in an Age of Revolution. New York: W.W. Norton & Co., 2005.

4. Lavoisier A-L, Pierre S, Marquis de La Place. Memoir on Heat, 1780. In: Fulton JF, Wilson LG (eds). Selected Readings in the History of Physiology. Springfield, IL: Charles C. Thomas, 1966:127-132.

5. Beddoes B, Watt J. Considerations on the Medicinal Use of Factitious Airs, and on the Manner of Obtaining Them in Large Quantities. Bristol: Bulgin and Rosser, 1794. (Available in Google Books)

6. Jay M. The Atmosphere of Heaven. The Unnatural Experiments of Dr. Beddoes and His Sons of Genius. New Haven: Yale University Press, 2009:292.

7. Bert P. La Pression Barometrique: Recherches de Physiologie Experimentale. Paris: G. Masson, 1878. Translated by Hitchcock MA and Hitchcock FA and published as Barometric Pressure: Researches in Experimental Physiology. Bethesda: Underseas Medical Society, 1978.

8. Acott C. Oxygen toxicity. A brief history of oxygen in diving. SPUMS J 1999; 29:150-155. (A publication of the South Pacific Underwater Medical Society.)

9. Balentine JD. Pathology of Oxygen Toxicity. New York: Academic Press, 1982:12-13.

10. Crapo JD, Barry BE, Foscue HA, Shelburne J. Structural and biochemical changes in rat lungs occurring during exposure to lethal and adaptive doses of oxygen. Am Rev Respir Dis 1980; 122:123-143.

11. Klein J. Normobaric pulmonary oxygen toxicity. Anesth Analg 1990; 70:195-207.

12. Deneke SM, Fanburg BL. Normobaric oxygen toxicity of the lung. N Engl J Med 1980; 303:76-86.

13. Clark JM, Lambertsen CJ. Pulmonary oxygen toxicity: a review. Pharmacol Rev 1971; 23:37-133.

14. Fracica PJ, Knapp MJ, Piantadosi CA, et al. Responses of baboons to prolonged hyperoxia: physiology and quantitative pathology. J Appl Physiol 1991; 71:2352-2362.

15. Caldwell PRB, Lee WL, Schildkraut HS, Archibald ER. Changes in lung volume, diffusing capacity, and blood gases in men breathing oxygen. J Appl Physiol 1966; 21:1477-1483.

16. Davis WB, Rennard SI, Bitterman PB, Crystal RG. Pulmonary oxygen toxicity. Early reversible changes in human alveolar structures induced by hyperoxia. N Engl J Med 1983; 309:878-883.

17. Loiseaux-Meunier MN, Bedu M, Gentou C, et al. Oxygen toxicity: simultaneous measure of pentane and malondialdehyde in humans exposed to hyperoxia. Biomed Pharmacother 2001; 55:163-169.

18. Sinclair SE, Altemier WA, Matute-Bello G, Chi EY. Augmented lung injury due to interaction between hyperoxia and mechanical ventilation. Crit Care Med 2004; 32:2496-2501.

19. Barber RE, Lee J, Hamilton WK. Oxygen toxicity in man. A prospective study in patients with irreversible brain damage. N Engl J Med 1970; 283:1478-1484.

20. Fläring UB, Rooyackers OE, Hebert C, et al. Temporal changes in whole-blood and plasma glutathione in ICU patients with multiple organ failure. Intensive Care Med 2005; 31:1072-1078.

21. Selenium in Intensive Care (SIC): results of a prospective randomized, placebo-controlled, multiple-center study in patients with severe systemic inflammatory response syndrome, sepsis, and septic shock. Crit Care Med 2007; 35:118-126.

22. Pincemail J, Bertrans Y, Hanique G, et al. Evaluation of vitamin E deficiency in patients with adult respiratory distress syndrome. Ann NY Acad Sci 1989; 570:498-500.

23. Marik P, Khangoora V, Rivera R, et al. Hydrocortisone, vitamin C, and thiamine for the treatment of severe sepsis and septic shock. Chest 2017; 151:1229-1238.

24. Tierney DF, Ayers L, Kasuyama RS. Altered sensitivity to oxygen toxicity. Am Rev Respir Dis 1977; 115:59-65.

25. Patterson CE, Butler JA, Byrne JA, Rhodes ML. Oxidant lung injury: intervention with sulfhydryl agents. Lung 1985; 163:23-32.

26. Kosower NS, Kosower EM. The glutathione status of cells. Int Rev Cytol 1978; 54:109-160.

27. Martensson J The effect of fasting on leukocyte and plasma glutathione and sulfur amino acid concentrations. Metab 1986; 35:118-121.

28. Smith LJ, Anderson J, Shamsuddin M, Hsueh W. Effect of fasting on hyperoxic lung injury in mice. Role of glutathione. Am Rev Respir Dis 1990; 141:141-149.

29. Register SD, Downs JB, Stock MC, Kirby RF. Is 50% oxygen harmful? Crit Care Med 1987; 15:598-601.

30. Bos KDJ. Diagnosis of acute respiratory distress syndrome by exhaled breath analysis. Ann Transl Med 2018; 6:33.

31. Müller-Wurtz LM, Kiefer D, Knauf J, et al. Differential response of pentanal and hexanal exhalation to supplemental oxygen and mechanical ventilation in rats. Molecules 2021; 26:2752.

SECTION 3

What Now?

What is the new oxygen paradigm?

14

"Fundamental progress has to do with the reinterpretation of basic ideas"

Alfred North Whitehead (1861 – 1947)

This book focuses on the destructive side of oxygen, and proposes that the human body is designed to limit exposure to oxygen, which limits the risk of oxidative tissue injury. This is contrary to the popular notion that the human body thrives on oxygen, and it challenges traditional beliefs about how the body is designed, how we die, and how certain patient populations should be managed. Some of these perceptual changes are included in Table 14.1.

The relevant information that supports this new "paradigm" is summarized in this chapter. The clinical implications of the paradigm are presented at the end of the chapter.

RELEVANT FEATURES

The Cardiorespiratory System

One of the ingrained concepts in the "oxygen mythos" is the notion that the heart and lungs are dedicated primarily to the delivery of O_2 to the tissues. This is discounted in Chapter 1, which includes the following information:

1. The ventilatory system is designed to control the elimination of CO_2.
2. Cardiac output is controlled by venous return, which suggests that the elimination of metabolic waste products (e.g., CO_2) is more important than O_2 delivery.
3. Any given change in cardiac output has a much greater influence on CO_2 removal than on O_2 delivery (see Figure 1.3 on page 10).

These observations indicate that *the heart and lungs are concerned more with eliminating CO_2 than delivering O_2*. This is a reflection of the relative abundance of CO_2 over O_2, as shown in Table 1.1 (see page 6). This difference is explained by the physiochemical properties of these gases; i.e., whereas O_2 does not readily dissolve in

TABLE 14.1   Changing Perspectives about the Human Design

1. The principal function of the heart and lungs is not O_2 delivery, but the transport and elimination of CO_2.

2. The principal function of hemoglobin is CO_2 removal, not O_2 delivery.

3. Hemoglobin holds O_2 from the tissues, since as many as 50% of the hemoglobin molecules never release O_2 into the tissues.

4. There is an oxygen-poor environment in tissues, and aerobic metabolism is designed to operate in such an environment.

5. Attempts to enhance tissue oxygenation with O_2 inhalation and RBC transfusions elicit countermeasures designed to maintain the oxygen-poor environment in tissues.

→ 6. All of the above features are designed to limit exposure to oxygen, because oxygen and its reactive derivatives are destructive molecules, capable of lethal cell injury.

water (plasma), CO_2 enters into a chemical reaction with water that produces carbonic acid (see Equation 14.1), and this reaction creates a "sink" that accommodates large volumes of CO_2. This reaction identifies CO_2 as an acid (a volatile acid), and this makes the lungs the major organ of acid excretion (see page 7).

Hemoglobin

Another ingrained feature of the "oxygen mythos" is the perception that hemoglobin is a dedicated vehicle for the delivery of O_2 to tissues. This is addressed in Chapter 2, which offers the following information:

1. The mass of circulating hemoglobin is 2.5 times greater than the mass of the heart, yet 25-50% of the circulating hemoglobin molecules never release O_2 into the tissues.
2. The large size of the hemoglobin pool is due to the fact that

it also is involved in the transport and elimination of CO_2. In this role, hemoglobin serves as a buffer for the carbonic acid generated by CO_2. The buffer capacity of hemoglobin is more than six times greater than the total buffer capacity of all plasma proteins (see Table 2.2 on page 23).

3. The volume of CO_2 transported by hemoglobin is three times greater that the volume of O_2 transported (see Table 2.3 on page 24).

As is the case with the cardiac output, *hemoglobin is more involved with CO_2 transport than with O_2 transport*. Furthermore, to accomplish the task of CO_2 transport, hemoglobin serves as the major buffer in the bloodstream. The involvement with CO_2 transport gives hemoglobin a much greater role than O_2 transport.

Plasma Bicarbonate

The buffering role of hemoglobin has implications for the perception of plasma bicarbonate as a buffer. This is explained using the reaction that generates carbonic acid (H_2CO_3):

$$CO_2 + H_2O \leftrightarrow H_2CO_3 \leftrightarrow H^+ + HCO_3^- \qquad (14.1)$$

This reaction occurs primarily in red blood cells (where the enzyme carbonic anhydrase is located); the H^+ is then buffered by hemoglobin, and the HCO_3^- moves into the plasma in exchange for chloride ions (see Figure 2.3 on page 23). This means that *the plasma HCO_3^- is a reflection of CO_2 transport, and is not a primary buffer*.

Tissue Oxygenation

The centerpiece of the new oxygen paradigm is the paucity of oxygen in the tissues, which is a reflection of the relative insolubility of O_2 in aqueous fluids. This is demonstrated in Chapter 3, and the information in this chapter can be summarized as follows:

1. An average-sized, healthy adult has less than one liter of total-body oxygen, and 98% is bound to hemoglobin. As shown in Table 3.2 (see page 32), the total volume of O_2 in all the tissues of the body is only about 14 mL (i.e., about one tablespoonful), and there is only about 3–4 mL in cells (i.e., less than one teaspoonful).

2. Aerobic metabolism can continue at PO_2 levels of 1 mm Hg and even lower (see the section on "Critical PO_2" on page 31).

This information shows that *there is normally an oxygen-poor environment in tissues, and especially in cells, and aerobic metabolism is designed to continue in such an environment.* The paucity of O_2 in tissues explains why the heart, lungs, and circulating hemoglobin pool are not as concerned with O_2 delivery as generally perceived.

Man as a Microaerophile

Humans are traditionally classified as "obligate aerobes," which are organisms that require oxygen to survive and must live in an oxygen-rich environment. However, from the standpoint of our functioning parts (i.e., our cells), we are more akin to "microaerophilic organisms," which are organisms that require oxygen to survive, but live in an oxygen-restricted environment because they are poisoned by oxygen. This distinction may help to correct the perceived importance of promoting tissue oxygenation.

Tissue O_2 and Survival

The notion that an oxygen-poor environment in tissues is the normal state of affairs seems diametrically opposed to the traditional belief that an oxygen-poor environment in tissues (i.e., tissue hypoxia) is a common cause of death. This discrepancy is addressed in Chapter 4, and the following information is considered relevant:

1. The perception that inadequate tissue oxygenation is a common prelude to death is based largely on studies that use an increase in plasma lactate levels (hyperlactatemia) as a marker of anaerobic metabolism. However, there are several pathological conditions where hyperlactatemia is aerobic in origin (see Table 4.1 on page 43), and one of these conditions is sepsis, which is one of the leading causes of death worldwide.

2. The emerging consensus is that increased lactate production in conditions of metabolic stress (e.g., exercise and sepsis) is aerobic in origin, and that lactate serves an additional source of energy (equivalent to glucose oxidation) in times of need.

Excluding studies that use hyperlactatemia as a marker of anaerobic metabolism, *there is no evidence that inadequate tissue oxygenation (anaerobic metabolism) is the final common pathway in the death of aerobic organisms.* In fact, as described later, the *presence* of oxygen may be responsible for the death of aerobic organisms.

Efforts to Promote Tissue Oxygenation

Considering that the tissues normally operate in an oxygen-poor environment, efforts to promote tissue oxygenation are often unnecessary and can be harmful. This issue is addressed in Chapters 5 and 6 for two popular interventions aimed at enhancing tissue oxygenation: oxygen therapy and RBC transfusions. The following observations are relevant:

1. Oxygen therapy is aimed at increasing the arterial PO_2, while RBC transfusions are aimed at increasing the hemoglobin and hematocrit levels, and there is no evidence that either of these goals is accompanied by an increase in tissue oxygenation.

2. Oxygen therapy and RBC transfusions both elicit countermeasures designed to protect the tissues from unnecessary increases in oxygenation. Oxygen therapy promotes systemic vasoconstriction, while RBC transfusions increase blood viscosity; both of these effects are impediments to blood flow, which will limit or erase the expected increases in O_2 delivery to the tissues.

The existence of countermeasures that oppose attempts to increase tissue oxygenation is a testament to the importance of maintaining a low-O_2 environment in tissues. This is an "intelligent design"; i.e., *maintaining an oxygen-poor environment in tissues is advantageous because it limits the risk of oxidative tissue injury* (see next section).

Destructive Nature of Oxygen

The advantage of limiting exposure to oxygen is known to anyone who uses tightly sealed plastic containers to keep food fresh. Oxygen disrupts organic molecules and decomposes organic matter, and this destruction is enhanced *in vivo* by the production of "reactive oxygen species" that are capable of lethal cell injury.

Hormesis

Reactive oxygen species (ROS) are not always our enemies; i.e., during "normal metabolism," they can participate in a number of physiological responses. Only when ROS production is accelerated (e.g., the inflammatory response) do they become a source of tissue injury. The condition where low doses of a toxic agent can have beneficial effects is known as *hormesis*.

Scope of Oxidative Damage

The wide reach of oxidative tissue injury is demonstrated in Chapters 9-11, which describe the participation of ROS in the damaging effects of inflammation, radiation, aging, and age-related diseases. The participation of ROS in inflammatory injury deserves special mention because there are a multitude of diseases in which inflammation plays a major role (see Table 9.1 on page 124), including two of the most prominent and lethal diseases in modern times (cardiovascular disease and sepsis). Because of this, *oxidative injury deserves recognition as a leading source of morbidity and mortality in modern times.* (*Note:* The participation of ROS in neoplastic diseases is not covered in this book, but this involvement adds to the impact of oxidative injury.)

Mortality

The general belief that inadequate tissue oxygenation is the final common pathway for death is addressed in Chapter 4, which reveals a lack of evidence to support this belief. In fact, the most common cause of death in intensive care units is septic shock with multiorgan failure, where the organ failure is a result of inflammatory tissue injury, so oxidative injury is a more likely prelude to death than inadequate oxygenation. Stated another way, *death is more likely to be related to the presence, not the absence, of oxygen.*

CLINICAL IMPLICATIONS

The new oxygen paradigm mandates an "oxygen-protective" management strategy, where there is a shift in emphasis from promoting tissue oxygenation to reducing oxidative tissue injury. The components of this management strategy are listed in Table 14.2. This strategy is particularly relevant for the care of acutely ill or seriously ill patients, who have the highest risk of oxidative injury.

Oxygen Therapy

The current use of O_2 therapy is not based on tissue O_2 needs, and is excessive (see Chapter 5). The following changes are recommended to reduce the excessive use of oxygen:

1. The current threshold for O_2 therapy ($SaO_2 < 90\%$ or $PaO_2 < 60$ mm Hg) should be lowered, because it is not the threshold for impaired tissue oxygenation. In fact, the threshold for O_2 therapy corresponds to only an 8% decrease in the arterial O_2 content, while the threshold for RBC transfusions corresponds to a 64% decrease in arterial O_2 content (see Figure 5.2 on page 59). (This not only shows that lower levels of arterial oxygenation can be tolerated, it also shows the arbitrary standards of O_2 therapy and RBC transfusions.) Lowering the

TABLE 14.2	Oxygen-Protective Management

1. Shift the emphasis from promoting tissue oxygenation to reducing oxidative tissue injury.

2. Reduce the excessive use of O_2 therapy and RBC transfusions by adopting a more reasoned approach to these interventions.

3. Abandon the use of plasma lactate as a marker of anaerobic metabolism.

4. Maintain antioxidant protection.

5. Develop a measure of unopposed biological oxidation for patient care.

threshold for O_2 therapy is an important step in reducing the excessive use of oxygen.

2. Because oxygen-induced vasoconstriction can erase the benefit of an increase in PaO_2 or SaO_2 (see Figure 5.5 on page 66), the following measures are recommended, when possible, to gauge the efficacy of O_2 therapy:

      a. Cardiac output

      b. Central venous PO_2

The cardiac output measurement will determine the influence of O_2 therapy on O_2 delivery (see Equation 5.3 on page 65). If this measurement is not possible, then the central venous PO_2 will be helpful; i.e., O_2 therapy should increase the central venous PO_2 if the arterial O_2 delivery has increased (see Figure 2.2 on page 20).

Measuring O_2 Consumption

A measure of the whole-body O_2 consumption (VO_2) represents a more reasoned approach to O_2 therapy; i.e., a normal VO_2 indicates that tissue oxygenation is sufficient to support aerobic metabolism, and O_2 therapy would not be necessary.

RBC Transfusions

The current use of RBC transfusions is not based on tissue O_2 needs and is excessive (see Chapter 6). The following is advised as a more physiological approach to RBC transfusions, and one that should reduce the frequency of transfusions.

1. The use of hemoglobin and hematocrit to guide RBC transfusions should be abandoned.

2. A better guide for RBC transfusions is the oxyhemoglobin saturation difference between arterial and central venous blood ($SaO_2 - SvO_2$). This is normally about 25% (indicating that 25% of the hemoglobin molecules have released O_2 into the tissues), and an increase to 50% represents the limit of compensation for anemia (see Figure 2.2 on page 20). Therefore, an ($SaO_2 - SvO_2$) of 50% can be used as a "transfusion trigger."

3. As described for O_2 therapy, a measure of the whole-body O_2 consumption (VO_2) could be used to determine the need for RBC transfusions; i.e., a normal VO_2 indicates that tissue oxygenation is sufficient to support aerobic metabolism, and RBC transfusions would not be necessary.

Plasma Lactate

Probably no measure has created more misperceptions about tissue oxygenation than the plasma lactate level. Hyperlactatemia has been the traditional marker of anaerobic metabolism, and a sign of circulatory shock, but (as described earlier) hyperlactatemia is often aerobic in origin.

Abandoning lactate as a marker of anaerobic metabolism will not only reduce the number of unnecessary and counterproductive attempts to promote tissue oxygenation, it will also reduce the number of ICU admissions.

Maintaining Antioxidant Protection

Attention to maintaining antioxidant protection is supported by evidence that antioxidant depletion is common in conditions associated with oxidative injury (see Table 12.2 on page 170), and it is almost universal in critically ill patients. The antioxidants that deserve attention (which are described in Chapter 12) include *glutathione* (the major intracellular antioxidant), *vitamin E* (the antioxidant in cell membranes and lipoproteins), and *vitamin C* (a scavenger of reactive oxygen species, and helps regenerate vitamin E). Antioxidant support is also provided by *selenium* (a cofactor for glutathione peroxidase) and *thiamine* (provides NADPH to keep glutathione in the reduced or active state). Monitoring and replacement of antioxidants is advised in conditions associated with oxidative injury (see Table 9.1 on page 124), and especially in critically ill or malnourished patients.

Glutathione

Monitoring the glutathione status is difficult because only a small fraction of glutathione is present outside of cells. However, glutathione has a rapid turnover rate, and deficiency is expected in seriously ill or malnourished patients (see Figure 13.3 on page 190). Exogenous glutathione is not appropriate for replacement therapy because it does not readily enter cells. However, N-acetylcysteine (NAC) is a glutathione precursor that readily enters cells and has proven effective for glutathione support in acetaminophen overdoses. Although the effective antioxidant dose is not known, an NAC dose of 600-1,200 mg twice daily is safe to use. (NAC is described on page 174.)

Hyperoxic Lung Injury

Attention to antioxidant protection is especially important for preventing hyperoxic lung injury in ventilator-dependent patients, because mechanical ventilation increases the risk of hyperoxic lung injury, and antioxidant depletion is common in these patients (see pages 187-190). Since glutathione is an important antioxidant in the lungs, the empiric use of glutathione replacement with NAC seems wise in ventilator-dependent patients, regardless of the O_2 requirement.

Comment

Although antioxidant therapy is hampered by uncertain treatment regimens and limited bioavailability (see pages 173-176), attention to maintaining antioxidant protection is necessary to combat oxidative tissue injury. Much more experimental work is required to develop more effective treatment regimens. Liposomal drug delivery has improved antioxidant bioavailability and efficacy in animal studies, but liposomal formulations are not routinely available for clinical use. Targeted therapies like this seem to be the future, and should be guided by measures of oxidative injury rather than clinical outcomes.

Monitoring Oxidative Injury

A measure of unopposed biological oxidation is necessary for any management strategy aimed at reducing oxidative injury. Several methods have been used experimentally, including the detection of lipid peroxidation products in plasma, urine, and exhaled breath; the detection of DNA strand breaks (comet assay) and oxidized guanine residues in urine; and assays of oxidized protein carbonyls in plasma. There is also an assay to assess the oxidizing power of plasma. However, none of these assays are routinely available, or approved, for patient care.

It is imperative to develop a measure of oxidative stress for clinical use, because focusing on the dangers of oxidation is the next great step in patient care.

Appendix

OTHER BOOKS OF INTEREST

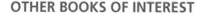

Detailed Texts

1. Halliwell B, Gutteridge JMC. *Free Radicals in Biology and Medicine*. 5th ed. Oxford: Oxford University Press, 2015.

   This is the traditional reference text for oxidative stress: an 800-page tome written by two pioneers in the field, that includes a wealth of information about oxidative stress in health and disease.

2. Sies H, ed. *Oxidative Stress. Eustress and Distress*. London: Academic Press, 2020.

   An ambitious text (with over 100 contributors) that includes a systems approach to oxidative stress, and emphasizes the difference between physiological and pathologic oxidative stress (eustress and distress, respectively).

3. Banerjee R, ed. *Redox Biochemistry*. Hoboken: John Wiley & Sons., Inc, 2008.

   Written by biochemists, this is a relatively compact text (285 pages) that covers all the relevant redox reactions in biochemistry.

4. Jacob C, Winyard PG, eds. *Redox Signaling and Regulation in Biology and Medicine*. Weinhein: WILEY-VCH Verlag GmbH & Co, 2009.

   This book includes 19 chapters (from 37 contributors) that cover the participation of reactive oxygen and nitrogen species in physiological control systems and aging. Provides a more balanced look at oxidative stress.

5. Armstrong D, Stratton RD, eds. *Oxidative Stress and Antioxidant Protection*. Hoboken: John Wiley & Sons, 2016.

   This book includes chapters on the role of oxidative stress in a wide variety of conditions, including ones that receive little attention, such as hearing loss, infertility, and schizophrenia.

6. Foote CS, Valentine JS, Greenberg A, Liebman JF, eds. *Active Oxygen in Chemistry*. New York: Blackie Academic & Professional,1995.

   An informative text on oxidation in nature and industry that requires more than a passing acquaintance with chemistry.

General Interest

1. Lane N. Oxygen: *The Molecule That Made the World*. Oxford: Oxford University Press, 2002.

   This is a wonderful book, full of information, wit, and insights, that is reminiscent of a Carl Sagan book. Like Sagan, the author (Nick Lane) has an authoritative background (in oxygen biochemistry) and the ability to captivate an audience.

2. Canfield DE. Oxygen: *A Four Billion Year History*. Princeton: Princeton University Press, 2014.

   This is a very readable book about the origins and control of atmospheric oxygen, written by an ecologist who peppers the narrative with his personal and professional experiences.

3. Walford RL. *Maximum Life Span*. New York: W.W. Norton & Co., 1983.

   A book with valuable insights about longevity, written by one of the early investigators of the longevity benefit associated with fasting.

4. Waldman J. *Rust. The Longest War*. New York: Simon & Schuster Paperbacks, 2015.

   This book focuses on corrosion and its impact on society. Of interest because it highlights the impact of oxidation outside the body.

The Discovery of Oxygen

1. Jackson J. *A World on Fire. A Heretic, an Aristocrat, and the Race to Discover Oxygen*. New York: Viking Penguin, 2005.

   A very readable history of how Joseph Priestley (the heretic) and Antoine Lavoisier (the aristocrat) contributed to the discovery of oxygen. The author has the eye of an historian for the social and political milieu of the time.

2. Bell MS. *Lavoisier in the Year One: The Birth of a New Science in an Age of Revolution*. New York: W.W. Norton & Co., 2005.

   An entertaining account of Antoine Lavoisier's role in the birth of modern chemistry (including his work with oxygen), and the tragic impact of the French Revolution on Lavoisier and his science.

Index

Page numbers followed by "f" indicate figures and those followed by "t" indicate tables.

209